ECSTASY & **AGONY**

The manic can see no problem;
the depressive can find no solution;
but all this is nullified by the powers of lithium . . .

ECSTASY & AGONY

LIVING WITH MOOD SWINGS

David Grounds MB, BS, FRACP, FRANZCP
and
June Armstrong B App Sc (Occ Th)

A LOTHIAN BOOK

A Lothian Book

Lothian Publishing Company Pty Ltd
A division of Thomas C. Lothian Pty Ltd
11 Munro Street, Port Melbourne, Victoria 3207

First published 1992

National Library of Australia
Cataloguing-in-publication data:

Grounds, David.
Ecstasy and Agony.

Includes index.
ISBN 0 85091 520 1.

1. Manic-depressive psychosis – Treatment.
2. Manic-depressive psychosis – case studies. I. Armstrong, June 1943- . II. Title. (Series: Lothian health guide).

616.895

Edited by White Kite Productions
Cover design by David Constable
Typeset in Sabon by MacKenzies
Printed in Australia by The Book Printer

FOREWORD

One of the most memorable television programmes I have ever watched was many years ago and it involved Spike Milligan. I remember the show not for Milligan's hilarity, but because he was profoundly depressed. It was a side of his personality the outside world had never seen and the revelation was troubling. He had agreed to come on air and talk about his mood disorder, along with a few other famous people who were willing to 'come out' and discuss their hitherto hidden disability. I said the revelation of seeing this renowned and normally energetic comic hardly moving and finding it difficult to speak was troubling. That was not because of any stigma; the feeling was of empathy and wanting to help.

It is a tragedy that at the end of the 20th Century it still requires guts to admit to others that you have a mental illness. Sometimes it takes a lot to admit it to yourself and the process of seeking help is often one of emerging from isolation. This book makes sense of bipolar mood disorder, or manic depression as it used to be called. By placing the stories of people who have experienced mood disorder alongside vital information, the authors help people with the condition and their families make decisions, feel more secure and less lonely or helpless. People with mood disorder lead normal and often highly creative lives; thanks to modern psychiatry. It's just important to understand what's going on, what medical science knows at the moment and what treatments are available.

This book is a fascinating read for people seeking answers but uncertain where to find them; it's for families wanting to help someone they love; it's even for professionals who can learn much from the stories and the up-to-date material; and finally it's for people who may not have any direct 'need to know' but who care about the human condition.

Dr Norman Swan

CONTENTS

ACKNOWLEDGEMENTS

We would like to pay tribute to the eight people who have told of their experiences in living with mood disorder, often at the cost of reawakening painful memories. Without their courage this book could not have been written.

Ms Lindsay Image, a skilled clinical psychologist, contributed the section on cognitive therapy.

Dr David Ingamells, a consultant psychiatrist and psychotherapist for many years at The Melbourne Clinic, wrote the section on the role of dynamic psychotherapy.

Dr Andrew Stocky, Medical Director of the Mother and Baby Program at The Melbourne Clinic, contributed the section on lithium in pregnancy and post-natal psychosis.

Dr Brendan Holwill wrote the first draft of The Melbourne Clinic's guide to lithium, used as a basis for Appendix II. Mrs Kay Gibbons wrote the Guide to MAOIs, Appendix III.

The editorial skills of Sally Moss demonstrated the difference between believing one has a good command of the English language and knowing how to write a book. We owe her a great debt.

Jill Clark, Margaret Hackett, Mandy Lane, Helen Mock and Lois Shephard typed the early drafts of the manuscript but the major burden fell on Robyn Smith, who showed unfailing tolerance in the face of the authors' apparently endless amendments. Healthscope and the management of The Melbourne Clinic (a Healthscope hospital) generously allowed us to use their word processors to produce the manuscript, and to reproduce pamphlets prepared by David Grounds on behalf of The Melbourne Clinic.

Finally our respective spouses, Pat and Richard, sacrificed our companionship during the writing of this small volume. As a first-time-published author, one of us (DG) wishes to acknowledge the learning curve he has undergone — so much time for so few words.

DG & JA

Will you ever love me?

I woke up one morning
dreaming I was a goddess
floated high on a cloud
revelled in sex to excess

Found myself a whirlwind
spending sprees down the days
flights from imagined deities
brightly garbed to amaze

Mania, mania ran amok
gabbling through the hours
no relief; endless fears
within the hidden powers

I woke up one morning
dreaming I had no passion
dribbling down in mood
to harvest full depression

Found myself in misery
no sleep to soothe the way
wondering if my children
would be allowed to stay

Depression had its full
weeping through the hours
no relief; endless fears
within the hidden powers

If I let you down again,
will you ever love me?

Anna

INTRODUCTION

These times could be called 'The Age of Exposure'. In no other period in civilisation have we humans subjected ourselves to so much psychological investigation and exposure. Evidence of this can be seen in the proliferation of courses and groups, and in the wave of media publicity, devoted to open exploration of personal identity and the weaknesses and strengths of the individual. Everything — from infertility, birth, sexuality, disease and death to spirituality and mental and physical disability — is exposed in minute detail as we probe the private and intimate lives of the famous and not so famous. We have an apparently unquenchable thirst for any information on the body, psyche and soul of others that might help explain what makes *us* tick.

This wealth of information offers us not only greater self-understanding but also increased tolerance of individual differences. As a result we feel less shock and more compassion when faced with a range of life and death experiences. Interwoven with this tolerance is a widening trend to take full responsibility for ourselves.

One group of disabled people has, until recent times, been given little publicity. This group, about one person in a hundred, suffers from manic-depressive disorder — or, as psychiatrists now prefer to call it, bipolar mood disorder. This can be an extraordinarily scary illness which, if not treated, condemns the sufferer to a life of intermittent highs and lows, called mania and depression. Yet between episodes of illness, these people are able to function productively at home, at work and in the social sphere.

Many highly creative and famous figures have suffered from the disorder. Virginia Woolf, Teddy Roosevelt, Vivien Leigh, Ernest Hemingway, George Frederick Handel, Franz Schubert and Robert Schumann were among them. In fact, a study of well-known artists, writers, actors and musicians found that they experienced four times the expected rate of manic disorder.

Comedian Spike Milligan has identified himself as a sufferer of bipolar mood disorder, speaking openly of his need to be admitted a number of times to psychiatric hospitals for treatment of severe depression. He has also experienced mania: irritability, elation, wit, loquacity, extraordinary energy. Commenting on his own case, he once said, 'You get the pain much worse than anyone else, but you see a sunrise much more beautiful than anybody else.' Milligan has made a genius's contribution to comedy and writing, being most renowned as one of the Goons.

The actress Patty Duke has also spoken of her experience with this disorder, and more importantly, has described how, through treatment, she has been able to maintain sufficient health to continue being a productive artist.

This book aims to reduce fear and encourage tolerance of bipolar mood disorder and its treatment — not only by stating the facts but also by demonstrating the courage of the sufferers, caught as they are in a web not of their own making. Eight people have allowed their stories to be recorded here, and the spectrum of talents and abilities thus revealed defies traditional notions of mental illness.

Many former sufferers are doctors, tradespeople, teachers, artists, parents or scientists, successful in their various fields of endeavour and making valuable contributions to other human lives despite their own suffering. Others have made progress in a more personal, less public way. For all these people the restoration of balance made possible by diagnosis and treatment has enabled them to achieve far more than they, their families or even their psychiatrists had anticipated.

1

MOOD DISORDER — WHAT IS IT?

This book is about mood disorders. There is much in it which relates to depressive illness, including the type called unipolar depression. However, it concentrates on a special form of mood disorder which consists, on the one hand, of extreme euphoria (also labelled 'mania', or 'hypomania' when it is less severe), and usually, on the other hand, episodes of severe depression (commonly called 'major' or 'psychotic' depression).

About one person in one hundred and fifty will have an episode of mania during their lifetime. (More will experience the milder degree of illness — hypomania.) However, as many as one person in ten will experience at least one episode of depression sufficiently severe to warrant treatment.

For the lay person trying to understand mood disorder, one of the difficulties is that it is really only an exaggeration of normal experience. With most physical diseases, by contrast, there is a clear line between the normal and the abnormal; you either have cancer, AIDS, a fractured bone, and so on, or you don't. Nevertheless, there is a qualitative, as well as a quantitative, difference between normally elated and depressed moods on the one hand, and mania and major depression on the other. On the high side, the difference is like that between a glider soaring and a supersonic aircraft crashing through the sound barrier; on the low side, the difference is like that between being down in the dumps and sitting in a bottomless pit in near-Stygian darkness.

Bipolar and Unipolar Mood Disorder

Some people have only manic attacks, some only depression, but the majority experience at least one episode of a mood disorder of the opposite pole to their usual.

It is quite common for depression to follow a manic episode. In a smaller proportion of cases there is a manic episode after depression. Patients who suffer from either manic episodes or both mania and depression belong to the group classified as sufferers of bipolar mood disorder. If a person has depression alone it is termed unipolar mood disorder, though the family history may suggest that the disorder is a bipolar one, with mania yet to raise its head. The distinction is important because most psychiatrists would view unipolar depression as a different illness: it tends to start later in life, it is less often linked to a family history of psychotic disorder, and the treatment differs in some respects.

Bipolar mood disorder is marked by pathological mood swings from euphoria to despair, by spontaneous remissions, and a tendency to recur. In the intervals between mania and depression, mood and behaviour are usually normal. Unlike a significant percentage of people suffering from schizophrenia, the vast majority of people with mania and depression do not deteriorate intellectually but, if left untreated, the disorder can be debilitating.

Life for an untreated sufferer can be like a ride through a steep mountain range. Remissions and relapses can be spontaneous and unpredictable. Climbs to manic peaks can go on for months, and the episode itself might last for six months to more than a year if untreated.

Few sufferers have a continuous switchback ride, but the majority have more than two episodes. The intervals between attacks may be many years, or a few months. Some have cycles of regular length, relapsing every three or seven (or however many) years.

'Normality' and Disorder

In trying to understand mood disorder, it is important to be very clear about what constitutes disorder or illness in general. When we speak of disorder, we are referring to a change in the structure or function of the body or mind which, from accumulated knowledge, we can categorise as a significant departure from an individual's usual 'personality' or from the variations found in healthy people, and which will cause the sufferer to feel ill or unwell.

On most occasions it is easy to obtain a consensus that certain behaviours are a sign of illness. If someone chopped down trees because they thought it was God's will, or claimed to be the reincarnation of Jesus Christ, few would doubt that they had lost touch with reality and were in fact psychotic.

On the other side of the coin, former Wimbledon champion Pat Cash certainly deviated from the norm in being so elated that he clambered up to his family on the shoulders of spectators after his win in 1987, but in the circumstances it was regarded as an understandable reaction rather than disordered behaviour. Similarly, a prime minister or president who openly weeps after defeat at the polls may be an embarrassment to those with a stiff upper lip but would not be regarded as suffering from depressive illness.

There are some situations in which differentiation is not easy. A person of previously even temperament who suddenly exhibits high spirits and boundless energy may attribute this behaviour to a new-found faith, or diet, or relationship, when in fact he or she is heading for an episode of mania. People with bipolar mood disorder, particularly in the early stages, often show infectious enthusiasm which can draw others in, sometimes with disastrous results. A proposer of exciting business ventures who is on a 'high' can persuade others to give financial support, when calm assessment by an outsider would lead to the conclusion that the project is doomed to failure.

Traditionally, judging a condition to be a disorder has been left to the medical profession, although it inevitably depends on society's norms. In the present age, however, the issue of civil liberty is challenging the prerogative of the medical profession to decide who is 'ill' and who is not. This is particularly so with psychiatric disorders, and some of the challenges come from within the psychiatric profession itself. Thomas Szasz, an American psychiatrist, has suggested that psychiatric illness is a myth created by those in power (with the connivance of the medical profession) to control what is deemed by authorities to be undesirable behaviour.

A denial of the existence of psychiatric illness is not new. In the nineteenth century, asylums for the mentally ill were built well away from population centres so that society could ignore the one per cent of the population who suffered from chronic psychosis. Now that the custom is to discharge such patients from institutions, one way of coming to terms with insanity is to say that the illness does not exist.

Surely a healthier approach would be to accept that there are certain biologically determined disorders and that these require treatment (whether the patient recognises it or not) to restore well-being, safety and health to the sufferer, and, to a much lesser extent, because of the risk to the community if the sufferer is untreated.

At the same time, the concepts of illness, involuntary treatment and danger need to be constantly reviewed. Once, the policy in mental hospitals was: 'If in doubt, keep the patient in hospital.' Now it is: 'If in doubt, discharge the patient.' And this change brings important responsibilities with it.

Psychiatrists find it easy to draw up criteria for the extremes of bipolar mood disorder — mania on the high side and psychotic depression on the low side. And even the lay person has little trouble recognising hypomania, a lesser form of mania, and non-psychotic forms of depression.

The difficulties arise in deciding whether to classify as ill, or just temperamental, someone who is at times high-spirited, talkative, overactive, impulsive in business, prodigal with money and sexually promiscuous, and at other times withdrawn, lacking in energy and interest, unable to perform adequately at work or socially, pessimistic about the future and unable to be jollied out of this state.

The distinction is important in deciding whether treatment is desirable. If the subject and those close to them do not believe they are 'ill', they are most unlikely to accept a trial of treatment. Indeed, if they do accept treatment, they might well decide afterwards that they prefer the ups and downs to the steadying effect of medication, but at least they have had the opportunity to assess this effect.

If someone is deemed ill, is treated, and then loses the dominant characteristics of their personality along with the mania and depression, was their former self an expression of personality, or of a psychiatric disorder?

When we refer to someone's personality, all who know them usually understand what we mean. However when it comes to pinpointing personality in the context of illness, the issue becomes much more complex. Psychologists and psychiatrists speak about a person's personality as the fairly stable aspects of their behaviour, mode of thinking and feeling, and other mental characteristics. Departures from this pattern usually indicate a disorder.

Symptoms and Signs

A person in normal high spirits has balanced judgement, is in control of their state of mind, and will respond to any appropriate dampening of that mood caused by day-to-day events. Conversely, it is normal to experience a flat mood, often caused by adverse life situations. We have all felt depressed at some time and had to take stock of our losses, disappointments, plans gone wrong or other mishaps. This sadness is appropriate to the situation, is usually brief and responds to support from family and friends.

Both the manic and the depressive phases of bipolar mood disorder have a different quality, producing behaviour that is inappropriate, prolonged and unaffected by the usual support mechanisms. Sufferers of bipolar disorder veer from elation, hyperactivity and Napoleonic ambition to (usually) severe depression, with lethargy, slowed thinking and, often, delusions of guilt or worthlessness. In depressive phases there are also often physical effects, including loss of appetite and weight, severe constipation, changes in the texture of the skin and hair, and loss of strength in the muscles.

A patient's husband describes his wife's illness thus:

'Initially, Wendy was just in high spirits. She seemed to have unlimited energy, even after short periods of sleep. She talked much more than she usually does, and she was much more interested in sex — in fact, more than I could cope with. However, she then started leaving the house on mysterious ventures and, when she came home, she would pace around boasting of her hidden powers as a goddess. She seemed to believe she was omnipotent and was going to deliver the supreme child. She couldn't concentrate on tasks and her conversation was an unbelievable babble at times. At other times she was hostile and suspicious and would often talk to herself.

'There was so much more: a series of happenings which left us all wrung out. In the end, the police intervened after she had rung them three times, and we managed to get her to a doctor. She was in hospital for several weeks. When she came home,

MANIA UNBRIDLED ECSTASY (FULL BLOWN MANIA)

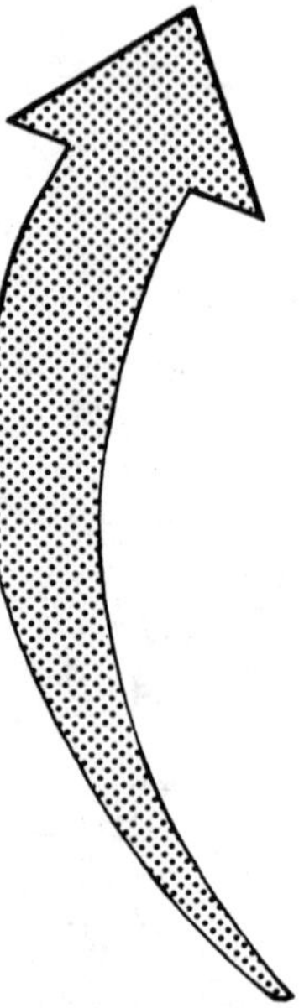

whirlwind activity
gross indiscretions
delusions of grandeur
absence of sleep
reckless driving
sexual indiscretions
shoplifting
flight of ideas
foolish business investments
elation
distractability
impatience and irritability
excessive spending
verbosity
decreased need for sleep
increased sociability
high spirits
greater energy

NORMAL MOOD (EUTHYMIA)

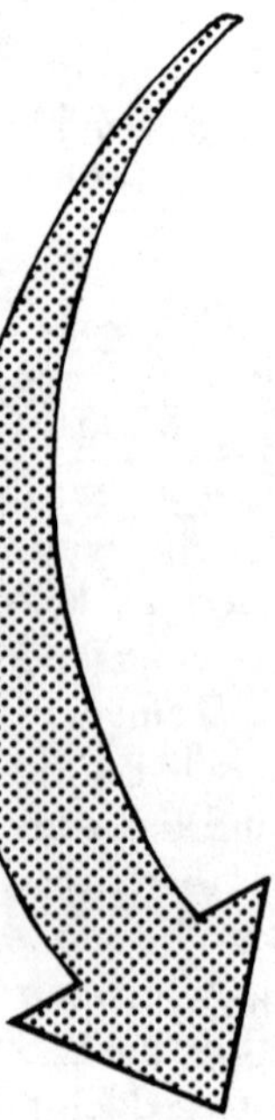

dispirited but can brighten up
disturbed sleep
slightly reduced appetite
sluggish
slowed thinking
reduced ability to enjoy usual interests
feeling of failure
weary of life
miserable and gloomy all the time
difficult to hold a conversation
self-accusations
better off dead
extremely despondent all the time
needs persuasion to eat
consideration of suicide
unable to do anything without help
emotionally paralysed
delusions of ruin or sin
explicit plans for suicide with active preparation

DEPRESSION THE PIT OF DESPAIR (PSYCHOTIC DEPRESSION)

instead of the overactive, elated person who went to hospital, we had a morose, agitated Wendy, unable to sleep and frightened to be left alone.

'She had been high in October and November and now, in January, she was depressed. We all wondered how we could continue adjusting to these swings, and for the children it was particularly difficult. They were quite distraught.'

Contributing Factors

It was originally thought that mood disorders were more common in the upper and middle social, educational and occupational classes, in contrast to the almost universal finding of an increased incidence of schizophrenia in lower class groups. However, more recent investigations have found no clear-cut relationship between social class and mood disorder.

While some psychiatrists of the psychodynamic (Freudian) school still regard psychological factors as being the major cause of bipolar mood disorder, most authorities today would say that such factors, particularly losses or events which represent losses, may indeed *precipitate* an attack, but, as it can also occur spontaneously, they are not true causes.

There are, however, certain factors which do have some bearing on the occurrence of mood disorder.

Personality

People who might be described as moody, and in whom periods of relatively high spirits alternate with periods of inactivity and being down in the dumps, are certainly more likely to develop the full-blown characteristics of severe mood disorder. For reasons which are not yet clear, the person with an obsessional personality who is conscientious, perfectionist and predictable is more likely to develop major depression than people with other personality traits, though not more likely to develop the bipolar picture of mania and depression. This does not mean, of course, that *all* people of obsessional personality will develop serious depression, or that they are the only personality type which does so.

The personality demonstrated by a person before the onset of illness will colour the clinical picture that emerges. When depressed, those who have been acquisitive of material goods are more likely to have delusions of poverty, and those who had a tendency to hypochondriasis are more likely to develop delusions of fatal illness. In mania, those who have always been less likely to conform with society's values are likely to be more outrageous in their behaviour during a 'high'. In other words, the illness exaggerates the sufferer's normal tendencies.

There is another side to the coin. People who have had strong personalities, standing up to the slings and arrows of outrageous fortune in their lives, disintegrate less under the onslaught of a depression.

Age

For physiological reasons which we will explore later, age has many influences on mood disorder. There is a tendency for episodes of depression to be more severe and frequent as age increases, and suicide is more common, even in situations where loneliness is not a factor. Mention has already been made of the blurring between major depression and dementia in the elderly, and of course both may be present in the one person.

It is also important to look at influences at the other end of the age scale. Although most adolescent sufferers present with the same features of mania or depressive illness that occur in adults, there are age-specific differences. Behaviour which can be ascribed to normal teenage turbulence — outbursts of severe loss of emotional control, hyperactivity and disturbed relationships — might be evidence of mood disorder and should probably be suspected as such if there is a family history of the illness. Similarly, the urge to leave home, or feelings of not being understood or approved of, withdrawal from the family, school difficulties and grouchiness might be features of a depressive episode.

Even professionals will have problems in assessing whether or not mood disorder is the cause of such behaviour. For this reason, it is better to err on the side of caution, and seek help even if it turns out to be unwarranted, than to allow the suffering to continue and to worsen. With dramatic increases in youth suicide in the Western world, families would do better to overreact than to underreact to mood swings observed in young people.

Gender

Of all people with depression, women are, statistically, twice as likely as men to have a mood disorder. (See page 137.) However, in bipolar disorder the female predominance is not nearly so marked. In surveys the ratios of women to men vary from 1.5:1 to 1:1.

Genetics

Although the tendency for bipolar mood disorder (and schizophrenia) to run in families has been observed for over a century, there has been ongoing argument as to whether this is nature or nurture or both — that is, whether the disorder occurred as a result of inheriting a faulty gene, or of growing up in a family where the previous generation contained sufferers, or a combination of both.

However, advanced statistical data and recent medical research (including studies of the incidence of the disorder in identical twins compared with non-identical twins) have thrown new light on the significance of genetic factors. The answer is even clearer thanks to the development of modern molecular biology and the discovery of the structure of DNA — the famous double helix which houses our genes and thereby determines our nature.

Using sophisticated scientific and statistical techniques, two medical scientists, Egeland in the USA and Mendlewicz in Belgium, have been able to discover the locality of genetic discrepancies in families with bipolar disorder, the former study finding it on chromosome 11 and the latter on the X chromosome. Other abnormal gene locations may yet be found.

Through these findings we now know that bipolar mood disorder is clearly due to disordered brain metabolism, and there are so many substances involved in the chain of reactions we call metabolism that a number of genetic faults could lead to any one disturbance in behaviour.

However, not all people who inherit the faulty gene suffer from the illness, suggesting that other factors, presumably environmental, also play a role in the development of the symptoms.

Mood disorder also occurs in people without a family history of the disorder, particularly those who develop the disease later in life, and while this still may be due to a spontaneous mutation of a gene, rather than a genetic defect inherited from previous generations, another possible explanation is that the disorder may arise from some disease which develops in the brain and causes genetic abnormality but which itself is not genetically determined.

Statistics are notoriously inaccurate in psychiatry, where

'head-counting' is so dependent on the experience, framework and biases of the observer; but we can be fairly certain that the number of so-called 'first-degree relatives' (parents, siblings, offspring) of a person with bipolar mood disorder who will themselves exhibit signs of the illness is somewhere between ten and twenty per cent.

The higher the number of sufferers in the family, the greater the possibility of handing on a faulty gene to one's children. The risk depends on a variety of environmental factors and the genetic lottery (only half of each parent's genes combine to form the fertilised egg, and we cannot know whether our half contains the faulty gene).

At The Melbourne Clinic we know of a family of three children all of whom developed the disease and two of whom suicided. On the other hand, some people with the disorder have many children, all unaffected.

Childbirth

It is increasingly recognised that women in any given age group are more likely to present with symptoms of a mood disorder in the year following the birth of an infant than they are at any other time.

The majority of the mood disorders exhibited are not related to bipolar mood disorder. The most common mood disturbance is that of 'baby blues' — a transient phenomenon which occurs before the fourth day post-partum and is associated with tearfulness, rapid change of mood, and anxiety. Often the mother reports crying without feeling depressed and therefore without knowing why. This phenomenon does seem strongly linked with hormonal changes, and occurs in up to sixty per cent of women giving birth.

Post-natal depression also commonly follows childbirth. Between ten and fifteen per cent of mothers complain of some depressive symptoms, with frequent complaints of difficulty in coping, constant exhaustion, tearfulness and a sense of failing in their role as a mother and a partner. Only a small percentage of these require psychiatric treatment, and most improve with support and encouragement.

However, there is a disturbance, puerperal psychosis, which does seem to be a mood disorder of a manic type. This disturbance, which occurs after one in five hundred births and usually presents within the first two weeks, is more common in women who have a strong family history of mania or who have themselves had an episode of mania or a previous puerperal psychosis. The new mother tends to present with a dramatic illness associated with an elevated but rapidly altering mood, confusion, a major inability to cope, and possibly hallucination and delusions. If she has had a previous puerperal psychosis, or a past history of a manic illness, she has a one-in-five chance of a recurrence with subsequent pregnancies.

There is some controversy as to whether puerperal psychosis is a mood disorder or whether it is a separate class of illness. The fact that it tends to respond well to lithium therapy (see page 68) indicates that it is probably a type of manic illness. Not only does treatment with lithium tend to result in a much speedier recovery from the illness, but the prophylactic use of lithium during the third trimester of the pregnancy and continuing use immediately after birth greatly decrease the chance of a recurrence of the psychosis in subsequent pregnancies. A recent clinical trial suggested that prophylactic use of lithium decreases the chance of recurrence to one in twenty-five (one-fifth of the usual probability).

Doctors generally believe that all drugs should be avoided during pregnancy if possible, particularly in the first three months, during which the foetal body and organ systems are developing. Some doctors think that, if a woman takes lithium in the first three months of pregnancy, there is a significant risk of abnormalities in the baby, particularly heart abnormalities. However, many psychiatrists believe that this risk has been overstated. They believe that, if the mother ceases lithium therapy before conception, the risk of mania or severe depression (and their consequences) outweighs the risk to the baby if the mother continues lithium.

Women with puerperal psychosis need inpatient care. In order to minimise the effect of the illness on the process of mother/baby bonding, the inpatient unit should have facilities for admitting the baby as well. There is a limited number of such units in Australia. The only one in the private sector opened at The Melbourne Clinic in 1992 and is staffed by a multidisciplinary team including psychiatrists, psychiatric nurses, midwives, paediatricians, a maternal and child health nurse, an infant psychiatrist, an occupational therapist and a social worker. Only such a broadly skilled team can provide the support needed by the mother and her infant.

Trigger Factors

A mood swing is sometimes precipitated by stressful life experiences. Depression can follow actual or symbolic loss; for example, the death of a family member or close friend, loss of a job or inability to get one, being uprooted from your home for any of a number of reasons, being burgled or burnt out, or experiencing a life-threatening illness or the break-up of a relationship.

Some stressors which result in a depressive episode are not so obvious or dramatic as those just mentioned.

Stressful experiences that can trigger a high include overseas air travel, being driven (or driving yourself) too hard at work, the onset of a new relationship, drug abuse, making a long-term commitment to another person (for example, through engagement), and childbirth.

Although a mood swing resulting from a loss is usually a depression, and the swing which follows a stimulating stressor is commonly a manic one, this is not always so; sometimes the direction of the swing is contrary to what would be expected.

Mood swing episodes are often not associated with clearly recognisable factors. Some are determined by the seasons of the year, and some just happen — 'When the apple is ripe, it will drop from the tree.'

The Physiology of Mood Disorder

The genes we inherit from our parents are present in every cell. Under their influence we develop the multitude of different types of cells that make up the body, all interacting in a system so complex that the most advanced computer is a simple toy by comparison. In the brain, electrochemical interactions control mood, as well as action, thought, memory, sensations, and so on. If we experience a glorious sunset the message is passed from the eye to the part of the brain that receives the image and on to our consciousness, or awareness. A further message then goes from that area to what is called the limbic system of the brain, which is concerned with mood, and we feel pleasure.

These messages travel down the nerve cell as a type of electrical phenomenon and when they reach the end of the cell which is adjacent to the beginning of the next cell they release one of many types of chemicals in the brain, which transmits the message between one cell and the next. The chemicals are known as neurotransmitters. A very large number have been discovered, and this makes it difficult to determine which causes what effect, but it is believed that those concerned with mood are mainly noradrenaline, serotonin and dopamine.

In episodes of mania or depression there are changes in the amounts of these transmitters within the limbic system, so that mood is artificially altered. Presumably this is because some switching mechanism goes astray and upsets the normal biological rhythm. There are many rhythms within the brain, the one most familiar to us being the rhythm of waking and sleeping. Another is the seasonal rhythm mentioned later in this chapter. All the drug treatments of depression appear to change the levels of the neurotransmitters to control the mood disorder until the faulty switching mechanism returns to normal.

Mood Disorder and Other Psychiatric Disorders

Schizophrenia

Problems often arise in differentiating between bipolar mood disorder and schizophrenia. Patients with mania commonly suffer some of the symptoms of schizophrenia, such as auditory hallucinations and delusions. Some patients' symptoms are in an intermediate position, and they receive a diagnosis of schizo-affective disorder; while a few patients clearly have both disorders, with different symptoms occurring in different episodes. Until recent years, it was the practice in North America to diagnose schizophrenia, rather than bipolar mood disorder, if any of the symptoms of schizophrenia were present. ('If there is a touch of schizophrenia, then the patient has schizophrenia.') This resulted in a lower reported incidence of bipolar mood disorder and a higher reported incidence of schizophrenia in the United States, as compared with Europe and Australia, which tended to go in the opposite direction. ('If there is a touch of mania, it's manic depressive psychosis.')

Increasing co-operation between psychiatrists worldwide has led to a more uniform approach to diagnosis, particularly when many people with a diagnosis of schizophrenia in the United States responded dramatically to use of the drug lithium, which is very effective in severe mood disorder and rarely helps in true schizophrenia.

Just as mania can be mistaken for schizophrenia, so can major depression if there are delusions present. If the delusions are in keeping with the mood, such as delusions of poverty or sinfulness, the distinction is not so difficult. However some people with psychotic levels of depression have delusions which are not in keeping with their mood, such as persecutory delusions.

In rare cases a patient might also have delusions that people can insert unwanted thoughts into their mind, or read their thoughts, or even control their thoughts and behaviour. As the treatment for the two disorders is different, lengthy observation and skilled judgement may be required so that the appropriate diagnosis is made.

Some psychiatrists find that a biochemical test, the dexamethasone suppression test (known as the DST), is useful in the differential diagnosis between schizophrenia and major depression, for the test is rarely positive in the former and very often so in the latter.

Dexamethasone is a cortisone-like substance which the patient takes in tablet form. When the pituitary gland in the brain detects its presence in the body it sends a chemical message to the gland responsible for producing the body's own cortisone, telling it to cut down production because it has been supplied from outside the body. In people who are well, production usually takes more than twenty-four hours to resume. In people with major depression, for reasons we do not yet understand, production of cortisone resumes much sooner. There is no evidence that a lack of body cortisone, or an excess, is itself a cause of depression. Rather, this test uses body cortisone as a *marker* of depressive illness, just as the level of sex hormone in urine is used as a marker of pregnancy.

Although there is argument about its reliability, many psychiatrists find the DST useful, especially in deciding when to reduce or cease treatment. If the test remains strongly positive, it is wise to continue the treatment.

Alzheimer's Disease

In the elderly, major depression is sometimes confused with Alzheimer's disease (the most common cause of senile dementia). Symptoms which are common to both include apathy, complaints of difficulty in concentration and memory, and disorientation. One patient in her eighties who developed this picture after fracturing her leg was diagnosed by the family doctor as being demented and was put on a waiting list for a nursing home. After she had spent some time in the nursing home, another doctor was called in to treat her, and it was only then that the original diagnosis was corrected. The second doctor recognised that a woman who, just prior to the fracture, had been preparing horses for the Royal Melbourne Show could hardly have developed sudden dementia. Mute, wasted and in danger of dying, she was quickly admitted to a psychiatric hospital for treatment. After a course of electroconvulsive therapy she made a full recovery.

Seasonal Affective Disorder

In the early 1980s, psychiatrists and biologists identified a mood disorder with a strong relationship to the seasons, which they named seasonal affective disorder (SAD).

Sufferers experience a type of depression in winter and hyperactivity in summer. Certain clinical features separate it from bipolar disorder, even though some people who suffer from the latter have depressive episodes in winter and highs in summer.

The winter depressions of SAD share with other sorts of depression a lowering of mood, energy, sexual drive and concentration, and social withdrawal. However, in contrast to those who suffer unipolar and bipolar depression, patients exhibit a craving for carbohydrates, gain weight, are tired (more so in the late afternoon) and have increased hours of sleep, sometimes sleeping more than twelve hours. By contrast, in the summer they often need little sleep, getting up at 4.00 a.m., bursting with energy and ready to start the day.

Some sufferers find that their mood lifts if they travel to a summer climate, only to relapse into depression on return to winter. Travel from a summer to a winter climate has the reverse effect.

Researchers believe the disorder may be linked to the level of production of melatonin, a hormone produced by the small gland which is situated near the base of the brain. The production of melatonin follows a circadian rhythm — that is, it ebbs and flows according to the time of day. During daylight hours the level is suppressed, increasing after sunset and reaching a peak at about 2.00 a.m. In people with SAD the elevated levels overshoot into daylight hours, and start rising earlier in the late afternoon.

Strong light suppresses melatonin production, and when sufferers from SAD sit in front of a battery of lamps for two to four hours a day and look into the lights for a second or so every minute, they gradually remit from their depression. However, after the light therapy is terminated, the improvement disappears and the condition steadily relapses.

Scientists are investigating the disorder and its relationship with melatonin, in the hope of finding the cause of the disorder and the basis of the improvement with light therapy. Light therapy does not benefit normal subjects or people suffering from unipolar depression.

Jet lag is a well-known phenomenon related to alterations in the circadian rhythms and recently light exposure has been recommended for this, too, to reset the internal clock.

Schizophrenia is not the only condition sometimes mistaken for mania. Medications such as cortisone and other steroids can trigger a manic episode, as can amphetamines. Antidepressant drugs can also cause a 'high' which may result in a person with unipolar disorder being wrongly diagnosed as having a bipolar one. If a person has a history of previous episodes of mood disorder, either mania or depression, or both, it is highly likely that the development of major depression is another episode in an ongoing disorder. Nevertheless it is part of the process of assessment to ensure that this episode is not due to some physical disease which may be treatable, such as an adverse reaction to medication or illicit drugs, to thyroid gland disorder, some types of anaemia or, occasionally, to cancer.

An illness inseparable from severe clinical depression can be caused by many medications, for example those prescribed for high blood pressure. Infectious diseases such as influenza, hepatitis and glandular fever may cause depression, as cancer can, even before it is diagnosed.

Alex

'I think my disorder was brought on by stress and my body chemistry.'

My family is intriguing. I had an aunt, my mother's elder sister, who suffered from a nervous condition. In those years, through ignorance, people didn't know what was the matter with her. She spent some time in and out of hospital. Her suffering was one where she couldn't open the front door if anybody knocked. She'd been hiding all the time, and I know that she was a constant house cleaner, always dashing around. You'd walk through the lounge and she'd be there with the carpet sweeper behind you, as though you'd made a hell of a mess. She may have suffered depressions and elations, I'm not sure... I know she used to go off to Royal Park now and again. But she had no children and she was sort of alienated from the family to a large degree. In latter years she seemed to mellow and Mum got back together with her again, and she didn't suffer from those traumas like she did in her earlier days.

I had an active, exciting family life as a child. My father's family were all league footballers with Fitzroy club. It wasn't until I was about fourteen that I started to excel in the field of running, and this was mainly from my mother's encouragement.

My mother was very loving. Dad was far more interested in my elder sister because of her sporting capabilities. It wasn't until I started to succeed in a bit of sport that I really became a person — I always felt second rate to my elder sister. She had also done better than I had done in primary school. But later I progressed well, and I won a scholarship in Form 4. Beyond that, when I started work I did very well, and I served an apprenticeship to the trade of electrical fitting. I got a couple of awards for scholastic achievement — both through the firm that I worked with and through the Apprenticeship Commission.

Right from the time when I was a child I've always been a very hyped-up person. I can vividly remember sitting underneath the kitchen table and singing my head off. Not that I had much notice taken of me, but I could always hype myself up. I had no problems in that regard. In my early teens, when I started getting interested in motor cars, I could stay up all night for days on end, just tinkering — putting cars together and pulling them apart.

I suffered from lack of concentration as a school student. I think it was just one of those things — I couldn't keep my mind on one thing for a particularly long time, and only when I found the subject areas that interested me did I start to do well.

Having served my apprenticeship I was very ambitious, and I wanted to become the foreman of the works where I was employed. I got within cooee of that, in so far as another fellow and myself were being groomed to take the job. After spending about nine months waiting on this situation, I decided that I would look elsewhere. From there I went to another firm where I got a grand opportunity in the way of lift mechanics, and became the first leading hand ever appointed with Johns and Waygoods. Within six years I'd paid off my house, drove the latest model Jaguar motor car, and didn't owe anybody a cent. I had to leave that particular firm. I got to the point of acting foreman with that company, and was offered a job as manager of a new branch in Tasmania. I refused that and I accepted another offer to go back to my old company. My job was to set up a service division within the company, with a further promise when this was done to advance to a sales engineering position, which I duly attained. I spent some ten years in that role, and enjoyed it immensely. But the company saw fit to divorce the operations in which I was involved, which was primarily automotive body building.

From there on I went into school teaching, where I've spent the last twenty years. I've enjoyed every moment of this time. But I suppose I find the frustration of administration overwhelming: the promotional opportunities that either do or don't exist, the manner in which curriculum is developed and implemented, and the needs that are there for the students — all of these things have got to have some relationship to one another. As far as I'm concerned, the authorities haven't come to the party. I don't feel that in my twenty years of teaching I've been able to contribute what I would really like to have done.

Early signs of my disorder began some seven years ago, and I think were brought on by stress and my body chemistry... I was teaching a fifth form at the college. We took in students who had failed Form 4 at any of the technical schools or high schools in the district, interviewed these folk and selected those we could handle. We agreed to take them on at Form 5 level. After a couple of years of this, I found that the pressure and the lack of support from the college itself just seemed to be getting me down further and further. I got to a point where I couldn't sleep. That wasn't so bad, but then, as time went on, my physical control of myself started to give out. I had a case of the shakes. My mathematical ability started to slip, and it just simply got worse and worse until one day I finally collapsed. Prior to that final collapse, incidentally, a friend of mine, whose wife was a doctor, diagnosed my trouble and dispensed me some Mogadon. That didn't help me one iota. It was just like taking Aspro. When I did finally collapse, my wife took me to a doctor, who referred me to a psychiatrist. But I was in no shape to do anything by that time.

I was actually quite depressed. Shades of grey was how I'd describe my mood. I'm quite sure that I was carrying out my job. I do remember that a very good friend in my department used to take me up and down to the tea room because, from the floor that I worked on, there was no way that I'd have found my way up... I must have been confused. It wasn't so much a mental confusion as a physical confusion. I've mentioned that my body seemed to be shaking all over, but the worst feeling that I had was like having a tin of worms inside me — my whole stomach seemed to be crawling. I used to force my fist into my stomach to try and stop it, and there was no way that this could alleviate the situation. A couple of days before I collapsed I can remember driving home from school, then walking some four kilometres to where my wife was working, to get her to help me. I don't know why anybody would want to do that, being weak and helpless as I was — why the mind said, well, we'll walk across and do this.

My family were most understanding — at first they couldn't believe it but, of course, eventually they had to. Having a doctor as a very close friend was quite a help. I think that it was really accepted that I was going to get better. It was just something that had come over me and it would duly go.

One of my very good friends with whom I spent three months of my long-service leave trip was most adamant, when the psychiatrist admitted me to the medical clinic, that my wife should get me out of that madhouse. It was only a place for 'dill-pots' and that type of thing. The unfortunate matter was that the same fellow had a nervous breakdown about three years ago, while chief of the vice squad in Melbourne, and he wouldn't have medical help. I suppose it took him another two years to get over that.

When I came home I can very vividly remember saying to my wife, 'I can't go on any further. Would you be all right without me?' She knew what I meant. I'm a keen shooter, I have a number of dogs, and those things are not new to me. I felt there was no way I could maintain the effort to stay on this planet as it was. I was suicidal. She was so shocked that I would contemplate doing such a thing that she was prepared to support me, no matter what or how. I guess the shame that I should contemplate doing something like that shocked us all. As it happened, I didn't attempt suicide, but it wouldn't have been difficult at all.

I was hospitalised and sedated. For about two and a half days straight I just slept. I was shut in a room and kept under surveillance. But I don't recollect anything. When I came out of it I underwent various tests and treatments in order to find out what was going to be of benefit to me. It was contemplated that I would have shock treatment, and at this point I was in no state to say yes, no or otherwise; but my wife was completely against that. The doctor then said, 'We can attack it other ways, but that would be the quickest way to get him over this problem.' We went through a range of different pills before my psychiatrist said that I would best be treated with lithium. My wife had different views again. She thought, 'This is a permanent treatment, but he doesn't have a permanent sickness.' I went back to work — within three and a half weeks of my first collapse. I suppose I had something like about four months back at work, and of course I crashed down again.

It was depression, and I was just slowly grinding to a halt, not able to carry myself in any way. At this point, my wife still resisted the suggestion of the lithium, thinking that, if she could take me away for a holiday for a few weeks, this might be the answer. So we hooked one of the caravans to the car and off we went to the coast. I can remember backing the car onto the beach. My wife didn't stop me but she wondered how in the hell we would ever get out of there. I was still pretty helpless by this stage, but I was able to go and buy a rope and tie it onto the van and get the car up on firm ground and haul it out. To me, that was a great achievement. Having actually done something was important because, all of this time I'd been away, I'd been fed and looked after and babied, and I didn't feel like I was getting anywhere at all. I do think it's important to feel some form of achievement in this recuperation stage.

My highs were interesting. On my long-service leave I

decided, with some persuasion from the policeman that I mentioned, to give up my lithium tablets. Less than four weeks later, we were on a dirt road in the Pine Gap area of the Northern Territory — crocodile country — and we were crossing a river. I thought to myself, 'Gee, that looks like good water.' It was about 7.30 at night, pretty dark, and I said to my wife, 'Let's get out and we'll fill the caravan with water. That looks good.' She said, 'I'm not getting out where those crocodiles are.' I became agitated, and told her she could go home — by plane, train or the bus, I didn't care how. Of course, she was very upset and was crying, and at this point I started to realise that this was in fact one of these highs that my psychiatrist had been talking about. Believe it or not I got straight back on my lithium and I suppose within the week I was back to something like normal. If I had not recognised that as being a high, it could have ruined both the holiday and my marriage.

When I'm on a high I wouldn't find it unreasonable to have sex with my wife every night of the week; whereas in my depressed state I might not want sex for say two or three weeks, and that's an obvious change of the health situation. I've never spent to any great excess, so I can't honestly say that I splurge and break the bank. But when I'm on a high I'm not particularly concerned about the other people. It's a great feeling... You think you can do no wrong, there's nothing that you can't do, and you just go ahead and do it, irrespective of others about you.

It must have been nine months before I agreed to take lithium. I had the first lot in hospital, in The Melbourne Clinic. The second time would have been about four months later, and my wife nursed me at home. She still resisted but finally gave in with regards to the lithium treatment. It wasn't until I was established on the lithium that I had any success. I commenced lithium treatment in something like 1980 and was on a stabilised programme within a few years. I can honestly say that I have not had any attacks since. But I can feel when I'm on a bit of a high, and I can feel when I'm on a bit of a low, and I would say that these highs and lows are more than those experienced by the normal person just going through the joys or disappointments of daily life. When I'm on a slight high I like to get all my exam papers written, do any jobs around the home, or complete something that I want to get out of the way. Whereas, when I'm on a low, every jolly thing, even getting the mail from the letterbox, is an effort. I can recognise these differences, but they are nowhere near the levels I reached before taking lithium tablets.

Restoration of my life would have come sooner had we not objected to the treatment. Oddly enough, to this day I still play games with my doctor. If he says two tablets, I take one and a half. If he says three I take two and a half, and it's only when I realise that things are not quite right that I revert strictly to his recommendation.

I consider myself very lucky, and fortunate. I'd have to say these problems have drawn my wife and me far closer together than I'd ever have believed possible, because the compassion that my wife has shown me during my illness is somewhat unbelievable. Not that anyone would wish to test a marriage by being afflicted with this disorder.

As far as my psychiatrist and I are concerned, I regard him very highly. I admire him as a man, and I can speak with him quite frankly without any reservations at all. For the best part of my life I've been the healthiest beast that ever drew breath and I've never taken any drugs of any sort. Having had this particular condition, I've come to accept that lithium is the only thing that keeps me going and functional. I realise that if I'd had a broken arm I'd have needed to have it set and repaired or whatever. My condition is such that I require lithium, and I'm quite contented and quite happy to take it. I don't say lithium has given me the opportunity to reach a higher level, but certainly it has enabled me to go on, because without it I would certainly not have gone on. There was only one way out and that was the back door. I'm now able to work and hold my place with my fellows, and my home life and relations with the rest of my family and friends are quite normal.

Sometimes I also take serepax, because I have occasional problems sleeping. If I've sat up till twelve o'clock or one o'clock in the morning marking exam papers, it is a little bit stimulating, and when I go to bed I can't sleep. Taking half a serepax enables me to get a good night's sleep and keep things in order. If I have a night without sleep it might run on for three or four nights in a row, and that starts to worry me. Sometimes I try to get to sleep without any medication, but I find that I have to revert to half a serepax. But I don't take a lot of them. I suppose I wouldn't take more than half a dozen in a month — I'm certainly not habitual with them.

I don't regard myself as being different from anybody, and I can perform all the duties that are required of me. I do a little bit more than that, too, in my job situation. I'm in the area of post-apprenticeship electrical mechanics and industrial electronics. There are something like fourteen of us teaching at the college. I was one of the foundation members of this particular area, and I've taken great pride in the fact that mostly anything that exists there I've either built or had a hand in building, in the way of equipment and experimentation and so forth. The school was used as a model for the building of other colleges throughout the state after we originally set it up, and it's gratifying to see that the work done in the early years is being duplicated at other colleges. Firstly, I think you need management skills, because before you do anything, of course, it's got to be thoroughly planned. Secondly, I think I brought to the college a high degree of hands-on skills in the electronics and electrical industries. My skills have not been affected by my disorder. I've been lucky in so far as the work that I've been in has given me a very wide breadth of experience.

Others at work know about my disorder. There were those who were sceptical, with the attitude 'He's had it, he's no good now', but I still find that those same people come for help and assistance and guidance when they are in a bother.

My ambitions are many. I certainly hope to see my family — my grandchildren, that is — grow up. I suppose I'd like to see them all turn twenty-one. Maybe that's possible, maybe it's not. But I have one big ambition in life: on my retirement I'm hoping to build myself an ocean-going yacht and I'd like to sail across to Samoa. Hopefully my wife will accompany me.

2

MANIA

Symptoms and Signs

Psychiatrists are in general agreement that, in order to diagnose an episode of disturbed behaviour as mania, the criteria laid down in the *Diagnostic and Statistical Manual of Mental Disorders of the American Psychiatric Association* should be met.

The manual cites the essential feature of mania as a distinct period when the predominant mood is either elevated, expansive or irritable, and this must be a prominent part of the illness and relatively persistent, although it may alternate or intermingle with depressed mood.

It must last for at least a week, and symptoms associated with the manic syndrome must be present, particularly an increase in activity, either socially, at work or sexually, or physical restlessness; an increase in talkativeness or pressure to keep talking, a flight of ideas from one subject to another or the feeling that thoughts are racing, inflated self-esteem or grandiosity amounting to delusion; a decreased need for sleep, distractability — that is, responding too easily to unimportant or irrelevant external stimuli; and an excessive involvement in activities with a high potential for painful consequences which is not acknowledged — for example, buying sprees, shoplifting, sexual indiscretions, foolish business investments, or reckless driving.

In some patients the delusions and hallucinations of grandiosity show themes of inflated worth, power, knowledge, identity or special relationships to a deity or famous person. Other patients suffer delusions or hallucinations that are purely persecutory, with beliefs that their thoughts are being controlled.

Even when people are on a high, brief concurrent episodes of depression can occur. One patient, a bank manager, recalls how, between episodes of excessive buying and visiting dozens of people at all hours of the night (with some of whom he had sexual relations), he felt very weepy and low. He also had some insights into what made him feel low, but he still did not realise he was ill. The hyperactivity often has a disorganised, flamboyant or bizarre quality — for example, dressing in colourful or strange garments, wearing excessive poorly applied make-up, or distributing money and advice to passing strangers. The increased talkativeness can take the form of jokes, puns or amusing irrelevancies. The capacity for normal speech might be lost, with a string of words taking its place. Speech might become theatrical, with dramatic mannerisms and singing.

The flights of ideas cause a nearly continuous flow of accelerated speech with abrupt changes from topic to topic, usually based on distracting associations. This can make the speech disorganised and unintelligible.

Due to the inflated self-esteem or grandiosity, a person might phone up or talk to people, offering all sorts of advice, from how to run the United States to organising birth control for the community. A book might be started, music composed, inventions designed. The person might lay claim to special talents but be unable to complete the work. (Many talented people have produced brilliant works prior to being acutely manic, and have been able to go on and complete them after recovery. But the manic phase submerges these talents.)

Distractability also shows itself as rapid changes in speech or activity as the person responds readily and quickly to all sorts of irrelevant stimuli such as background noise, signs, people, pictures, books, and so on.

Not all of these features of mania appear overnight. The picture is usually one of increasing severity, from the presence of an unusually good mood, greater energy, talkativeness, social contact and spending to grandiosity and intrusive, domineering behaviour, and ultimately reaching the uncontrolled stage of frenetic and erratic thinking.

Psychotic Symptoms

When the brain functions in such a way that normal reasoning is lost, and hallucinations and delusions occur, the sufferer's condition is termed *psychotic*.

Lynne, thirty-five, suddenly saw all car number plates as codes in a conspiracy against her, with white cars holding highest rank. She believed these were her funeral cars and that death was inevitable if she could not avoid them. Naturally this created great gripping terror and she drove wildly trying to avoid her persecutors, taking side tracks and detours at a dangerous speed. She also had an overwhelming sense that she was to give birth to a holy child, then die. A game of hide and seek ensued whereby she dropped into public phones to call strangers and tell them of the great events impending. Her delusions about the child were so strong that she approached a man to be the father and made all sorts of preparations in her bedroom.

Hallucinations occur when the person in a manic episode replaces perceptions of reality with imaginings. They may be very vivid and cause the person to lose sight of the real world. Flashes of visions; imagined voices and sounds; and strange, acute smells and tastes can occur. There might even be hallucinations of being touched by people, animals or insects.

The voices commonly heard are from persecutors, or deities believed to be asserting control. For example, a sufferer might hear the voice of God saying they are a chosen person, or someone else saying they are unfit to stay alive. These voices are very disruptive to normal daily living, all the more so once the person hearing them realises that the messages received cannot be trusted.

Barb, forty, saw vivid 'pictures' of her 'Master' and heard him giving instructions to leave her home before it was destroyed. She raced with her children to a neighbour's house and rang the police. They promptly rang a doctor, who arranged for her treatment.

John, forty-two, did not have such a safety net. He 'heard' voices telling him to die, for he was a wonderful sacrifice to the gods. A psychiatrist had given him medication but had not admitted him to hospital. He was free to lie on a bed, talking loudly all the time, sometimes laughing and sometimes crying, and swallowing a large proportion of his tablets. He recalls: 'I could vividly see, smell, hear messages, and only on looking back could I begin to sort out fact from fantasy.'

Delusions are belief systems which are not in touch with reality and are a sign of severe mental disorder. They have a powerful hold over the sufferer and can therefore be very disruptive or frightening. The content of a delusion is strongly influenced by the person's past and present experiences. Delusions are sometimes sudden and fully developed, and immediately believed by the person who experiences them.

One patient suddenly believed that all people wearing white were out on the streets to see her, a chosen person. Another believed people were hunting him. A patient reading a newspaper article about an aeroplane disaster immediately felt responsible for it, whilst another believed he was a Nobel-prize-winning professor.

Hypomania

When a person experiences mood elevation but there is no clear loss of touch with reality — that is, there are no delusions or hallucinations — the disorder is diagnosed by psychiatrists as *hypomania*.

Sufferers show many of the features of mania, such as elation, excessive talkativeness, distractability, irritability, impatience, impulsiveness and an impressive energy. Although they would benefit from psychiatric treatment, impaired judgement often prevents them from realising this, and current State government policies have tightened the criteria for compulsory admission. As a result, many families watch a hypomanic relative destroy the very basis of domestic harmony, their only weapon emotional blackmail, which is usually lost on the grandiose patient.

Fortunately people who have suffered from mania in the past, and have sometimes been committed to hospital, often recognise what is happening and, with the salutary experience of past humiliation to aid their limited insight, seek treatment.

People with lesser degrees of hypomania may in fact benefit, rather than suffer from their increased energy and ambition. But insight and control are the key. We probably all know people who are risk-taking workaholics and on social occasions are the life of the party. They always seem to have the accelerator pressed to the floor. It is only when a major depression interrupts this long-term hypomanic episode that anyone who knows them considers the possibility that their 'high' was not just a personality trait, but an abnormal state that meets the criteria of illness.

Altered Libido

Mood influences sexual desire and activity. Libido increases in hypomania and mania, and decreases in major depression, causing strained relationships, at least until the sufferer is diagnosed as ill. Swings between one extreme and the other are particularly difficult for a partner to accept. Since people in a manic or hypomanic episode tend neither to discriminate about sexual partners nor to consider taking precautions, they not only endanger their marriages or other relationships but they also risk contracting sexually transmitted diseases.

The impulse to demand constant sexual activity with partners or spouses, and to go further afield into promiscuous relationships, is beyond their control. It is a relentless driving force linked with high energy and extroverted behaviour which runs its course unless the person is hospitalised and treated.

A patient of ours, Anna, fell prone to this problem. She was overseas at the time, and can now recall her adventures vividly. However, at the time she had little insight into what she was doing. At one stage during a party she attracted a lot of attention with her vivacity, and in a rear bedroom had intercourse with three men. Another time she travelled with a man met casually and together they had so much sex that she was exhausted.

Richard

'When I was manic, I felt that I was quite sane and other people were not quite on the ball.'

Around 1965, in Sydney, I was diagnosed as mentally ill. I did some silly things and my father flew up and brought me back to Melbourne. I didn't know what I was doing, but I was deranged. That was the first indication that there was something wrong, but I wasn't diagnosed as being manic-depressive. I was diagnosed as having a nervous breakdown. The 'manic-depressive' tag wasn't put on it till years later.

My first signs of illness would have been in my last year of school, which was 1964. I had trouble with exaggerated elation towards the end of that year but I just put up with it. I thought it was just part of living. I left school in September and failed matriculation.

I was... sort of in limbo, I guess you could call it. I was

still conscious of doing the right things, but then I'd get very hyped up and do things that I wouldn't normally do. I had a feeling that I was a bit different, and I thought I could do things — godlike — which weren't normal.

I can remember parts of one episode. People were sort of respecting me, driving down the road and looking, and I'd think 'they're coming to pay homage', as though I was part of an upper cult that everybody was coming into... as though we were one and that sort of thing.

I was told my mother had the same disorder. Once, when we were coming over Sydney Harbour, I said to my father, 'There is a Russian submarine.' I can't recall that but Dad picked it up because Mum had been going through the same sort of thing... At that stage Mum didn't really know what she had either; she thought it was something she had inherited from her mother.

You can go from really high to really low. The depression side of it was frightening but I certainly wasn't frightened when I was manic. I confronted people when I was manic. In Sydney I think I hit somebody because they didn't say 'Good morning' or 'Good evening' or something like that. And that was actually the culmination... When that accident happened the police were called in, and somebody must have called a doctor. He must have recognised the fact that I wasn't behaving normally. So, rather than charge me, he notified my father, who came up to Sydney and got me. He took me to hospital in Geelong.

That was about April 1965. I was in a padded cell for about an hour. I remember climbing out of the window, and being helped down and returned to the cell. I can't remember exactly how long I was in hospital the first time. I have been in hospital five times. I was given sleeping pills and I think major tranquillisers, and that was it. Each time.

I found it good because others were sick, too, and there is a sort of mateship in hospitals when people are getting better. But everything got boring after a week or so.

It didn't dawn on me until after I'd had treatment and so forth, what I'd actually done. It was always very hard to take, afterwards, in a depressing way. I always felt there was a cycle of highs and lows, and that sufficient pressure from external events could trigger a bout of one or the other. For example in situations when I have been under pressure, and feeling a great need to succeed, I have collapsed.

Each time it happened to me, I was in different circumstances, so that I was mixing with people I got on really well with but who didn't know me very well. There were no real problems. I am talking of about five instances of mania over ten years.

After I was out of hospital in Geelong they sent me to Tatura and the mania came on again. I was doing excessive things, and laughing uncontrollably at relatively mundane happenings. I think I finished off that job by telling my boss well and truly where to get off. My father came and got me again.

I worked with the Stock Association for another three or four years, and then I went to Mount Gambier. Here I had a manic attack. But that manic attack was low key, compared to the first two. That was in October 1974. I had increased my smoking and drinking, and behaved with overactivity. I was up at 4.00 a.m. and restless. My speech was rapid and I was expressing anger at being dominated. This followed the birth of our second child.

I felt I had too much 'go' in me. I was working with some cattle dogs and felt that I had a calling from God to do this; in fact it was a gift. I thought there was some connection with my relatives' grand behaviour during the war. You can see how mixed up I was.

My wife tended to recognise there was something wrong, and I went to the GP and he put me in touch with a psychiatrist. My psychiatrist put me on sedatives which had a short-term effect, and then he put me onto lithium after I had another major depression.

The thing is, when I was manic, I felt that I was quite sane and that some other people were not quite on the ball. I can't honestly think of anybody saying I was really mad... I can remember once, at Tatura, going to the hotel and tipping beer on somebody who obviously was quite a well-known character in the town, and a few eyebrows were raised then.

I can recall driving a car into Melbourne and playing with the accelerator pedal, going fast and slow — in control but being stupid. I also had an affair... with a woman down in Portland... I lived and worked in Mount Gambier and we had a strike in Portland and I had to go down there and work for nine weeks. That was where I met her. She was pregnant, too. That was the sort of unusual thing that I would never contemplate during normal stages.

Also, when I was manic, instead of going to bed at 9.30-10.00, I might be drinking and playing records and going to bed at 1.00 a.m. and getting up at 6.00, hyped up and really looking for it. But that can only go on for a certain time, and then all of a sudden you just go too far and do stupid things. I'm probably lucky that I've been caught in each situation. It hasn't really got out of hand.

One thing that has haunted me over the years is that hardly anybody I've worked with has bothered to enquire after my health. This is probably a selfish attitude... they did not recognise that I was ill and that I wasn't in full control. It made a great deal of difference to me to have someone ring up and say, 'Well, hard luck, you've had a rough trot.'

Depression has probably been with me all my life, up until, say, ten years ago. I can always remember as a kid getting called depressed, and at that stage thinking it was just normal. Now, thinking back, I know that it wasn't normal. But I could get out of my depressive state by doing things, or thinking about things, that I really enjoyed doing... sometimes. I was morose, and probably finding it hard to get into doing things. Being a bit of a loner was part of it. I was guilt ridden because I've always tried to do what I thought was right.

I've experienced about six bad depressions. I think, if you've got this illness through your life, it may not be until you reach maturity that the swings start to become obvious. I learnt to live with it and accepted it as normal. Now I don't have that. But the worst depressions came after I'd had a manic high. I was treated with drugs — antidepressants and sleeping tablets.

I had ECT, as far as I can remember, only when I was depressed. I can't really recall having it for being manic. It was to bring me back to reality. It is really very simple as far as the patient is concerned. From memory, you are wheeled in to where the doctor is, you are given a needle to put you to sleep, and then you wake up in your bed, and you are normally given a piece of toast and a cup of tea. I don't know what the treatment does to your body but, each time I've had it, it has just brought me back to reality and given me a bit of a headache. I can't really pinpoint any other side-effects, although some have been expressed by different people. So

I've never had any fear and I can only say that... it's helped me. I'd only be guessing how many ECT treatments I've had. It's hard because each time I've been in for depression I've had ECT, but I don't know whether they gave me three or four or five sessions, or what. I could have had anything from 15 to 30 between 1965 and 1976.

It was certainly upsetting for my wife at the time, but she was very supportive and, although when she first met me she didn't know what my complaint was, she just treated it as something that had to be overcome. It must have been a worry for her, and it was a worry for me, too, because there didn't seem to be a cure. I look at myself as someone who has had a mother affected, and a grandmother, and a great-grandmother, who, at that time, had not been successfully treated. Fortunately, my being treated with lithium has meant that our marriage is in harmony. You could say it hasn't been affected, because our families are supportive. The marriage has been very stable and we've got three boys who are a joy.

I commenced lithium treatment in 1976 and have not had any attacks since then. I suppose originally I was on Lithicarb. I'm not sure what the pills were called, but I used to have three when I got up and three at night. I used to find they affected my bowel actions a bit. Then I was changed to Priadel. I have three tablets at night. I don't really feel any ill effects, except sometimes I get a bit of a thirst at night. Lithium has basically given me stability in living, because now I can plan ahead, and not worry that I'm going to do something stupid or go off on a tangent. It is a great feeling not to have in the back of your mind that you might... all of a sudden... crack up. I'm not excited that I'm on a drug and that I have to take pills continually, but to achieve the goal of stability, it's been a real winner.

I had an up-and-down life, I suppose, from age 18 to age 28... but I always had a goal, always knew what I wanted to do. I'm a farmer now. I've always had a goal to work on the land, and I've always had a job associated with the land. I've always enjoyed the jobs that I did, even though I've failed some of them.

Working for myself has certainly been a big help. A rural atmosphere is very conducive to health. Even though it is a lot of hard work, it is certainly not the same as working in the city, in offices. There is stress with it. You have got to meet specifications and things as much as any other job. But being your own boss — and I am my own boss now — certainly allows you to do what you want to do instead of having someone else looking over your shoulder. It has certainly helped me, but, by the same token, I've had to be a self-starter and not inclined to take things too easy.

At present we run three properties. We've recently bought the third property in Toora, and to do that we're selling another property. Our aim is to breed cattle on the Toora property and fatten them at Warragul. The aim is to build the breeding herd up to about two hundred (at the moment we've got about a hundred) and sell the steers, or bullocks. So we breed beef cattle and we also fatten them, and at the moment we've taken on agistment cattle. I suppose the three places cover about four thousand acres, so that keeps me fairly busy. I'm responsible for the three places because I haven't got anybody working for me. I get casual labour for jobs I haven't got time to do, and also I've got the three boys who help when I can catch them. At the moment it's fairly tough because we are in the throes of selling one property, and we've also got to keep our eye on Toora where we've got nobody working. I've got to spend three or four days out of every seven up there, which means travelling between the two places. But it's a good life; I wouldn't swap it for quids.

My ambitions are to improve the property at Toora to as high a level as we can, plant trees, improve the pastures, that sort of thing. We're putting in a vineyard of twenty acres, and I've also got to do a little bit of work on that. There won't be a winery here as such, as grapes take three or four years to bear fruit. For a start, the fruit will be sold to other vineyards. Then, hopefully, it will go into our own wine with our own label. That's quite some ambition.

MAJOR DEPRESSION

Although some people with bipolar mood disorder suffer only episodes of mania, most at some stage have an episode of major depression. Some patients with a strong family history of mood swings in both directions suffer only from depressive episodes.

Symptoms and Signs

Episodes of depression can arise in a setting of normal mood, or follow one of elevated mood. They might occur very suddenly or, more usually, develop over a period of a week or two.

Some people don't even acknowledge that they feel depressed, which may seem surprising, but words are, after all, only symbols for our experience and if a person cannot match their state of mind with the symbol 'depression', it should be no more surprising than if a colour-blind person cannot distinguish between two colours. People who do not recognise their state as fitting the word *depression* might use or recognise other terms, such as *dejected, despondent, gloomy, despairing, helpless* or *hopeless*. Of course, most sufferers do recognise their depressed mood for what it is — more than the feeling of disappointment we might experience when our favourite football team loses. It is a pervasive mood, hanging like a grey blanket over them all day, though one of the characteristics of depressive illness is that it is usually worst when the sufferer first wakens in the morning and it improves through the day.

The symptoms of major depression occur on two levels — physical and mental — with some merging of the two.

Physical Symptoms

Amongst the physical symptoms there is nearly always a disturbance of appetite, overwhelmingly in the direction of appetite loss. Some people continue to force themselves to eat, but describe the taste of food as like cardboard or plastic. Weight loss usually occurs, and is sometimes severe if the illness is not recognised and treated early. In the minority of cases, where appetite increases, weight gain is often significant.

Headache is very common but often not reported unless it is specifically asked about, as the other symptoms are so distressing that the headache has a lower priority in the hierarchy of complaints.

In the profoundly depressed phase of bipolar mood disorder most people show little sign of activity, their limbs often ache and feel heavy, and they are sometimes unable to rouse themselves from bed. Terms used to describe this feeling of energy loss include exhausted, spent, all in, pooped or whacked. Sufferers often overlook the need to eat, and to drink fluids. The situation becomes more critical if they are living alone and/or have an uncaring family.

Sexual appetite also suffers. In both men and women there is a loss of spontaneous interest in sex, and an inability to respond to sexual stimulus.

Other physical symptoms include constipation, hair that is dull, lifeless or needs more frequent washing, and dry or scaly skin. Facial appearance alters, often with dramatic differences evident in photographs taken before and after successful treatment.

Major depression also affects vision. Patients often describe the world as drab or grey, and by this they do not only mean that it is without pleasure, but also that the colours have changed. The ability to be visually aware of the world is also affected. Many severely depressed patients perceive their surroundings only up to two or three metres away. One patient, as he started to recover, commented favourably on the photograph behind his psychiatrist's chair. He was amazed when told that it had been there all the time.

Mental Symptoms

For many depressives, particularly those who have always had a tendency to hypochondriasis, changes in bodily function can contribute to an increased preoccupation with physical symptoms, which in turn becomes a psychological symptom. At times this morbid introspection reaches a delusional degree, with people convinced they are suffering from cancer, or that their bowel has shrivelled up to a non-functioning string.

In addition to delusions related to sinfulness and health, there is commonly a delusion of poverty. This seems to be more common in those who are actually more affluent than the average, who come to believe that their successful businesses are failing and that they will be made bankrupt. (As with mania, the delusions are usually linked to the sufferer's life circumstances; but here they are inverted.) A man who was knighted for his work in the public sector, and who was very wealthy, had to be certified because he was convinced that he could not pay the twenty-dollars-per-day gap between the private hospital fee and his hospital insurance rebate; nor would he return voluntarily to the public institution to which he had previously been sent on certificate for a similar bout of psychotic depression.

The tendency to shoplift, which was mentioned as a symptom of mania, also occurs quite commonly in people suffering from severe depression, but for different reasons.

People suffering from mania or hypomania steal because they believe they are above the law and enjoy the thrill, and in any case they think they are too clever to be caught. The position of the depressed patient who shoplifts is very different. They feel they are bad and should be punished, and they are often looking for evidence to prove their worthlessness. In shops they steal in such a way that they are highly likely to be apprehended, and this is in fact what they hope for. Sometimes, because of their difficulty in thinking, they do not always describe their motivation in such clear terms, but the evidence is fairly clear. They rarely steal anything for their own use, and commonly steal objects which are of no practical value to their family. Furthermore, they express a sense of relief when they are apprehended. Depressed patients who shoplift are most often women, perhaps because women are usually the shoppers in the family, though there might be other psychological factors involved.

In men, exhibitionism (exposure of the genitals), can also occur during a depressive illness, for similar reasons.

In most people suffering major depression, thinking tends to be slowed down, and the content of thought is usually fairly morbid, particularly during the early hours of the morning when most people with significant depressive illness find themselves lying awake. They usually fall asleep readily after going to bed but wake after three or four hours and toss and turn. At the other end of the spectrum, a few people with major depression sleep excessively long.

Other mental symptoms of major depression include difficulty in concentrating (which makes reading or even watching television arduous and often unproductive), and loss of interest in activities which are normally pleasurable to the person concerned. The combination of these two symptoms leads to indecisiveness, even over such humdrum matters as what to wear for the day.

Guilt of some degree is nearly always present in a major depressive episode. It is usually so prominent that it is not just a result of failure to carry out one's normal responsibilities. In fact, even if the depressed person draws on their limited energy reserves and is as productive as usual, they still feel they have failed. The basis of the guilt might extend from self-blame to believing that the illness is a punishment for past transgressions, or even feeling responsible for terrible things happening in the world. At this stage the sufferer has clearly lost touch with reality and is suffering from delusions.

It is not surprising that suicidal thoughts are associated with these feelings and thoughts. What is little more than a thought that life is not worthwhile can descend into a feeling that one would be better off dead and finally lead to actual plans for suicide, sometimes with the delusional belief that it will save loved ones from further suffering.

Fifteen per cent of patients who suffer from recurrent major depression commit suicide. Tragic as this is in a treatable illness, it is even more distressing when depressed mothers of young children kill their offspring before suiciding, in the mistaken belief that they are saving the children from a fate worse than death.

Some patients become agitated, with both mental tension and purposeless motor activity. This is more common in people with the unipolar type of depression. Physical symptoms of anxiety such as chest and stomach pain, palpitations and shortness of breath can mistakenly lead to a search for a physical cause of the illness.

Sometimes the agitation dominates the clinical picture and might mask the depression to such an extent that a diagnosis of anxiety disorder is mistakenly made. Australian poet Les Murray's severe depressive episode was diagnosed after he was unable to board a plane to travel overseas because of agitation and anxiety. He responded to a course of 'sanity and mental balance tablets', as he calls his antidepressant medication.

Stewart

'I didn't want to believe I was a manic-depressive.'

It is difficult to say when my manic depression began. It may have been... certainly in the middle years of my married period, when I was in my thirties. But I didn't realise I was a manic-depressive until I was diagnosed.

I'm sure my father was a manic-depressive... I'm sure it's in the family, because certainly they had extremes of high and low. Father was an extremely domineering sort of person. I think there was a lot of repression there, really. I always regarded our family as being more strictly brought up than others. We lived in fear, really — fear of retribution for being naughty. Mother was a much quieter sort of person. I think she suffered quite a bit. She spent a lot of time trying to keep the peace. Certainly we had moments of happiness. But I think this repressive atmosphere in our childhood tended to make us submissive and took away our confidence.

I was always designated to be a doctor, and my brother was designated to be a lawyer — from the moment we were born. I wasn't too keen on the idea because my strengths lay in the humanities rather than the sciences. But I never ever did mention it; you were regarded as a failure if you didn't do what you were supposed to do. My father obviously placed us under a great deal of pressure. That radically affected my performance and gradings in school. Had I spent my energies in the things that I really liked I would have done extremely well. I didn't do too badly, but my main interests were really history and literature and things like that, not physics and maths. I think overall my gradings were better than average, but they could have been top. I passed the equivalent of VCE; but, again, had I been able to spend my time on things I really enjoyed, there would have been a lot more success.

I was having episodes of depression by then. I was under a great deal of pressure. In my final year of school I did sufficiently well to get into a medical course... but I took a stand at that stage and opted to go into the family business, which was a disaster.

I then went into industry, becoming a company director and general manager. I'd done well at work, I had a very large circle of friends, and was popular. No problems getting on with people at all. I was excessively motivated, very demanding, a perfectionist. I set very high goals and managed to achieve them. But then the son of my business partner was going to be made a director and, frankly, didn't deserve a job in the company at all. So I took a stand, and that soured relations between the two sides. From that moment the job became difficult because I was suffering an internal battle as well as an external battle.

I had four children, all at private schools. I ran a holiday house, my wife always had a car, and she didn't work. The demands were well and truly met, and that meant a hell of a lot of hard work. Now, I don't know what you call normal. Sure, you come home tired and the kids can upset you and all the rest of it, and you snap at them. Whether that is normal behaviour or not, I don't know. So, for complex reasons, my marriage broke down and it was after that that I felt I experienced the symptoms of mania or depression.

I have had at least several phases of depression in my life, and several manias. During manias, I would be the life and soul of the party or whatever till all hours of the morning — fast speech and all the other sorts of symptoms you read about. I would go away on a holiday, throw a party, the classic thing. I would make rash judgements as far as business deals were concerned, and would get impatient. Then the depression came after you realised what you'd done.

I bought one business and I didn't show the solicitor the contract because I thought it would be fine. That's in court at the moment. I bought some land up in Cairns; again the same thing. I find that, during my manic state, my business judgement isn't affected as much as my capacity to engage cautiously in the business decision, if that makes sense. So, in fact, I was spending excessively. The outcome of this has been a lot of problems, but it didn't quite lead me to bankruptcy.

Constant spending became a compulsion of mine. As I said, the other dangerous aspect about mania is that, during these episodes, you lose your sense of caution. You don't question things and you have no fear. Of course you are so vulnerable because people you are doing business with aren't going to stop you and say, 'Hey, aren't you being a bit reckless?' They're going to take your money.

The unfortunate thing is that as far as my personal business is concerned, up until the manic-depression bit, I had done extremely well. I was worth a lot of money, over half a million. It was pretty hard to lose all that.

My wife is from the country. She really didn't like Melbourne, and I always had the fond idea that I'd like a farm. That certainly wasn't a manic-depressive thing, I enjoy rural things. Anyway I got the farm... I didn't do much physical work on it, but a lot of other stuff... The pressures of doing that and doing my job were enormous. Then, when things started to break down in my marriage, I felt an immense strain.

As far as I'm concerned, it was the breakdown in my marriage which really upset me, particularly when my wife — my ex-wife — had promised me that we would have at least twelve months' marriage guidance and declared after three weeks that the marriage was finished. That was three years ago. It's still very painful. It is not just the marriage break-up, it is the family break-up as well. The two younger children are in Ballarat with her. The two older ones are in Melbourne with me. Marital break down, manic-depression, changing jobs, losing a lot of money — I've had heaps of trouble.

I was never hospitalised because of mania. My first realisation of illness was during an extremely intense bout of depression. My children — the older children — were extremely worried so they took me along to the GP, who put me onto a psychiatrist. That was when I realised that the damage had been done. I still grieve. I think forgiving myself is the hard part. I don't blame anyone for what has happened. I think my ex-wife is extremely tough on me. She blames me.

Well the depression which hospitalised me was so intense I just couldn't do anything. I mean I'd literally sit down in a chair and that was that. I would just stay there all day. I was not very well. I would sleep through. I would sleep to escape rather than to sleep, if that makes sense. I tried to look reasonably tidy, but I wouldn't bother eating or about anything else. I didn't bother about conversing.

I was treated with lithium basically, and antidepressants. The other phases of depression that I had in my life were fairly mild compared to this bout. Depressions followed manic attacks.

I commenced lithium treatment about fifteen months ago. But I stopped it because, although I had been told by a specialist that I was a manic-depressive, I didn't want to believe it. Then I had more attacks of mania and depression.

I became increasingly manic. I'd re-established myself very successfully in the business of real estate. I'd made some bad decisions as far as employment was concerned after that. I got myself very well established in one particular agency and thought I'd do better at another one, so I changed. I thought I'd be able to get into off-shore money...

My colleagues didn't like it while I was manic. They didn't believe what was going on. I wasn't dismissed. I just decided I was doing so well in one particular area, I'd do even better in another one, without analysing the reasons for the success. After the mania and following depression I went to a smaller company — in fact, built it up...

After one bout of major depression I went back to my psychiatrist. I was re-established on lithium. My psychiatrist was terrific. I didn't think he'd see me, after my behaviour. By that stage I was fairly contrite. I think he has helped me an awful lot, just by putting up with me again. He is very understanding, and he realises I'm acutely disappointed in what has happened.

I can accept now that I am manic-depressive, but I don't have much self-esteem. I'm still feeling very mournful about what I've done. I am restoring order in my life now. I have met a lady I'm very fond of. I've got a fairly healthy relationship with my kids. It was very difficult to start with. Everyone was so unsure of me and felt a mistrust. People would look at me, and give me a quizzical look. Maybe I was sensitive, I don't know.

There are positive aspects. The real estate business I'm in now is a small agency, specialising in residential and investment. It has a business property section. The industry, as such, I find stimulating, but I haven't found the agency particularly invigorating. I feel I am under-achieving. I've made it difficult for myself because I started in it after I went out of the family company. The trouble is, if you make too many moves in a short time, people become suspicious. I was with the first company for twenty-eight years, and I left on very bad terms in the end. They wouldn't accept that there were medical reasons for my resignation. They wouldn't accept the manic-depression story, and as a result I went through a court action to get my superannuation, and that was tough.

There are certain qualities and needs in real estate work. I think the capacity to communicate is the Number One skill. Fortunately, despite all the rest of it, I have been able to communicate successfully. No one has realised I suffer mood swings, now I'm quiet. The funny thing is that perhaps a touch of quietness isn't a bad thing, because clients like to talk — they don't like someone talking to them all the time. I think, ultimately, lithium will enable me to reach a high level of performance in my work.

My ambitions are many; first of all to try and get out of the muddle I'm in; then to have a more successful career, help to raise the family, form a new relationship. I've got a lot on my plate.

(Since the interview Stewart has moved into a prestigious real estate and financial company, with considerably more responsibility and challenges.)

Lee

'I was relieved to find a reason for episodes I'd never really understood.'

My childhood is not an area I like to dwell on. I was born and brought up in Scotland. I was ten when war broke out and the children in Scotland were evacuated, so I was separated from my family for the next three or four years, and during that time my parents' marriage broke up. It was a very difficult time for practically everybody in England. We suffered a great deal. Children probably aren't aware of it as much as adults are, or they push it underneath and concentrate on snowballs or whatever interests them at that moment.

I attended a small village school in the north of Scotland which, rather than separating children at the age of eleven, took children through to the age of fourteen. Then those who were capable of it went on to what was known as the Academy. I stayed there until I was fourteen. I loved school. I was always in the top three in class and, without even thinking about it, took it for granted that I was going to get into the Academy and from there probably go to university. But, as I said, my parents separated. My mother went down to England and just around this time I was moved from the family I was staying with and billeted with an elderly couple — I was very unhappy there. I joined my mother. The education system in England was very different to that in Scotland, and it just wasn't possible for me to go to school any more. I had to leave at fourteen, which I found very distressing.

I worked at odd jobs until I was old enough to be accepted for nursing training. Well, I finished my general certificate. I enjoyed it very much, but... six months after I finished, at the age of twenty-one, I got married.

I had two children within sixteen months, and then had another one seven years later. For the first seven years I didn't go to work, because at that time a woman with children didn't go to work — she stayed at home to look after them. Whereas everybody now admits — or feels free to admit — to being bored by housework, nobody did then. That was anti-social. But I've never really liked housework, and I think I would have been a lot better off if I'd gone to work.

When my third child was born here in Australia, I had quite severe post-natal depression. That took a little while to get over. I don't know whether there is a connection between manic-depression and post-natal depression — I suspect that there might be because I have heard about it from other people. At the time I recognised this post-natal depression, but there were also good and sufficient external reasons for depression.

We'd only been in the country just under two years. We'd bought a very old house in the Dandenongs because that was the only place that we could find for which we could afford the deposit.

It was falling down — it was a one-hundred-year-old weatherboard. It had tank water, unmade roads, no mail delivery, snakes in the garden. I had two young children and the baby. I had trouble with the baby for the first six weeks or so... I couldn't breastfeed him. I'd breastfed the others and I felt terribly guilty about this. Guilt is part of depression.

Also, my husband had to go to Adelaide for a week on business with his firm at a time when I was just really sinking into this depression, and I think that made matters worse. I was left alone in the house. I couldn't drive, had no car, and was out in the sticks. For somebody who had been living in London with all mod cons, it was frightening.

It was dreadful. Terrible anxiety. I couldn't sleep at night. I had the baby in a crib by the bed, and I was in and out of bed to make sure that he was still breathing. I had obsessive-compulsive symptoms. I'd switch the kettle off, and then go back a couple of times to make sure I'd switched it off. I felt as though I was strung up so tightly — I knew I was sick. I said so to the doctor, who was a bit of a twit because he put me on Amytal (which in itself is depressing), but that was the only time I saw him. I gradually got over it.

I was just able to care for my baby sufficiently during this time. I had to; there wasn't anybody else there.

After a few weeks I got over it. I had a blazing row with my husband when he got home, since he didn't understand.

After that there were no problems for a number of years. The depressive episodes were the things that really caused trouble — for my family more than me. The highs I quite enjoyed... I got more done then because I was full of energy. I sometimes regret, in retrospect, that I don't get those charges of energy any more. But I didn't think I was depressed, at all.

The family knew that there was something wrong with me. I knew that there was something wrong with me. I didn't feel consciously depressed, but I knew I didn't feel well. I looked for a reason, and I could always find one. There was always this particular bug going around, or something. A virus or something. I would feel physically unwell, to the extent that I would go to bed for a while, because I knew I wasn't well. I think some time ago my psychiatrist said to me, 'That's quite right, you weren't well, but what was wrong with you was not what you thought it was.' As well as the depression, I used to get angry, because my husband couldn't understand that I was not well. I can remember saying to him many, many times, 'You don't understand' — which, of course, was true. Neither did I.

Since my younger son was three years old I have worked part-time, right through without a break, and I enjoyed that, but it was desperately busy — very, very busy and very tiring — and I never seemed to have time for self-indulgent things.

One year I remember getting the Monash summer programme in the mail, and I thought, 'That's nice, I'd like to do that, get right out, away from the house.' I wrote away and booked in for the music appreciation course. The secretary rang me and said unfortunately there had not been enough applicants and they'd cancelled it. Could she interest me in anything else? She read me a list of what was on, and one of them was creative writing. Now, I had no interest in creative writing at all, but it appealed to me more than the other ones, so I said, 'Oh, yes, I'll do that.' So I went, and there were about six other women and we sort of hit it off extraordinarily well. One of them was down from Geelong and was boarding at Monash and I thought, 'Isn't that marvellous!' So I went home that night and said, 'I'm not coming back for a week, I'm going to stay there.' I had a ball, I loved it. Now, that may have been a high. I was elated. I was having a marvellous time, thoroughly enjoying myself. I must say that I was chuffed during this experience to get very complimentary remarks on the bits of writing that we were forced to do.

But, you see, my highs really weren't a problem. I cite that as one because I think that I may have been slightly high to have had enough spunk to get up and do it, rather than stay around and worry about who was going to get meals for the next three days, or whatever, which was my normal pattern.

My highs were like a great charge. I didn't spend much money like some do. My husband and I had gone to see my psychiatrist and he asked whether I spent a lot of money when I was having these highs. My husband said, 'Yes.' My psychiatrist looked at him and said, 'What did she spend the money on — diamond rings, fur coats?' (This has become a family joke.) Tom said, 'Well, she bought me eight pairs of socks last week.' So, I don't really think I was ever guilty of that. But I did things that were out of character for me.

Another example was some time later. There was a lot of publicity being given to the fact that the Fire Brigade and the Ambulance Service didn't have the 'jaws of life' and the government wouldn't provide the money. For some reason or other I thought I would help with this, and I rang the Ambulance Service and told them what I had in mind. They were all for it. I went in there one day and went out with the crew in a MICA unit and also went to the recovery area of the Royal Melbourne Hospital. I was elated — I was getting on like a house on fire with this, getting along with everybody I met. Then all of a sudden I went blank. I thought to myself, 'Who the devil do I think I am?' I completely lost confidence, didn't take it any further which, as I say, fills me with shame.

So I really don't know whether highs gave me some sort of confidence that I didn't normally have to enable me to get up and do things which interested me anyway, but which I normally would cover with the washing and ironing and the shopping and all the rest of it. I wasn't frightened. I was enjoying myself, I thought I was doing something that was worthwhile, possibly selfish, but had a wonderful charge.

My husband thought it was great. He encouraged me. I told friends about the Monash episode and they thought it was great. I didn't tell anybody about the ambulance thing because I was a bit shy about it. When I ran out of steam and was starting to question myself, I was even less inclined to tell anybody about it.

Before I'd seen my psychiatrist for the first time, which must have been nine or ten years ago, I'd had several episodes of this feeling ill and going to bed for a week or a bit more, absolutely convinced I had the flu or some sort of viral infection or complete lack of dignity. I don't ever remember feeling deluded. I would get weepy, and accuse my husband of not understanding. But I went back to bed a lot, sometimes for days. It's a ghastly feeling.

I felt suicidal at one stage because of this terrible depression... but that was just one occasion. I frightened my brother once... I had been sleeping very badly, and one day I took some phenobarb and I went out like a light. My brother came in and sent for the doctor and made a fuss. But I hadn't attempted suicide, because the jar was half-full, I was just determined to get a good sleep. That was it. It frightened the hell out of them.

The first time, Tom got rather worried about me and bundled me into the car and took me down to my son-in-law who is a doctor. He talked to me for a while and then he rang a psychiatrist who told me I must go to hospital, because I was very depressed, I presume.

I've been hospitalised twice since in The Melbourne Clinic. But my psychiatrist treated me with antidepressants at first and they weren't really terribly successful. I used to get side-effects on them. But at the same time he was very reluctant to start me on lithium because of the possible side-effects and the continuing pathology that goes with it, so he held off on that. He eventually put me on lithium and I've been as right as rain since.

Each time I was admitted to hospital, I felt an overwhelming sense of relief. I was away from the pressure. I found it very interesting. It was 'time out'. I met a couple of people with whom I became friendly. I saw my psychiatrist every day, and did the usual craft and music and what have you. During these episodes I may have been in hospital for six weeks.

Like Tom, I was relieved to find that there was a reason for episodes that we had never been able to account for or understand. We remained together solidly right throughout. He's like a lot of other people; anything to do with mental illness floors him. But he is compassionate by nature, and it didn't throw him for long. He came to terms with it quite rapidly. We had rows before my condition was recognised or diagnosed; but since then, and certainly once I was stabilised on lithium, there haven't really been occasions for it.

I commenced lithium treatment at least six years ago — could be seven. I have not had any attacks while taking lithium. Until recently I would have said I haven't really had any side-effects. I get the odd tremor in my hand, but not often enough to worry about it.

The overall effect has been extremely good. It's hard to say because I have been well for such a long time now that I honestly don't think about it. The only time I have to think about it is when I have the lithium dose or go to see my psychiatrist. Apart from that, the lithium sits in the bathroom by the toothpaste and it is second nature — I just don't think about it. But it really has stabilised me.

I don't think of myself as a manic-depressive. From that point of view I accept myself completely. It doesn't worry me. I am a human with needs and interests like anybody else.

I'm a single-certificate nursing sister. I work in the field of psychiatry, oddly enough. One of the most important skills you need is the ability to listen — that's terribly important — empathise with people. I've always had these talents, skills and abilities — and I've just picked them up and begun again after I've been treated.

They don't know at work that I have suffered manic-depression. I tend to be private, so... I only tell people whom I know personally. It's not just manic-depression — I've also had cancer, but not many people know that either.

Just living normally has been a highlight for me since I became stabilised on lithium. Your confidence takes a tremendous battering. I don't have that worry now. I live quite happily, I want to continue to do so. I hope to go to Thailand next year. I have no large-scale ambitions — maybe that's the secret for success. It is a bit difficult to equate my life with ambition — I'm a quiet type really — go to work, come home, read a lot, have a garden, and a large hairy dog we're really fond of. Life is very full, really.

Tony

'I was simply obsessed with the fact that I needed to die.'

I think that there is a one-in-ten chance of a manic-depressive producing a child who will suffer the same disorder.

My father is dead now, but I have a feeling that he probably did get depressed, because he had a severe drinking problem, and it was never officially diagnosed. My sister gets depressed. I've never seen her suffering elation but she certainly has taken antidepressants and she's been in hospital from time to time. But I don't think she has good quality medical care. I think that makes a difference.

My daughter suffers already from eczema and migraines, which I understand are in the syndrome with depression. So... she may be one of those people. It doesn't worry me. Those are things beyond our control; I guess they have to be accepted.

As a child I went to a school for gifted children and I went through high school and did well. I attended university and got a Bachelor of Arts degree, and I always had top grades in everything. I went on to do a Masters degree, and I maintained good grades through that. As far as intellectual abilities go, that's something I'm pretty good at. I read a lot. I'm always involved in some new idea or other; it could be building a house, or gardening, or it could be just finding out new things.

I see films and appreciate them. I read lots of books... novels, poetry, short stories and plays, so my own cultural life is extended. Then, of course, being married to Susie (she has a degree in music as well as a degree in fine arts), we've had pretty good sessions, going out and seeing things, museums or whatever. The best part of the Masters degree is just understanding linguistics better. I really enjoyed it. I really became dedicated to the concept of learning.

Eventually I worked as a teacher for fifteen years. At first I tried hard to use every teaching method I could think of to encourage recalcitrant children to learn. I found out I don't like yelling. I found out that the kids can be brutal. I discovered that the educational system is uncaring. Also, I discovered that what I really enjoyed about literature, history, or whatever it was, wasn't shared by students, in general terms. There were always a few exceptions and that's one of the great rewards. I know some students who have done very well at HSC, and who have managed to get a good job through education, and that is nice. But on the whole it hasn't been a very rewarding fifteen years. In some ways I wish I hadn't done it because in the end it made me sick. In the end I had a breakdown and that's why I'm not working now. The cost to my friends and my family for the bad moods I got into, the anger, the constant frustration and my general unhappiness with my work was very damaging.

I didn't feel my breakdown coming, which I suppose is common for some people. There were lots of factors that fed into it. When I was teaching years ago, I was subject to a knife attack by an ex-student, which unsettled me a great deal. I guess the worst part was that I was set up by the kids in my HSC class who organised the fellow to come to the school when I was at a function. Anyway, some time afterwards I experienced a manic attack but I had no idea whether it had anything to do with that incident. I felt low and down in the dumps about it. I experienced constant shaking, crying and a sense of confusion. The feelings of depression were there in mild form, not in a severe form.

Eventually I went to another school and things just built up until finally I was crying all the time and I was just out of ideas, out of strategies, as to what to do. I got physical symptoms, a whole range of them. Eventually a colleague of mine said, 'Do you realise what you are doing?' I'd become violent that day at school. I said, 'What do you mean?' When he began pointing things out that he had observed, I started to cry, and everything collapsed at once. I just decided that I wasn't ever going back. I finally had to get medical reviews for WorkCare. The psychiatrist obviously believed what I told him, and I didn't hide any facts about having an illness either. I tried to explain that they were separate issues and that I knew the difference between them.

I think what happened is that the depression was evidenced pretty early in my life. All I can remember is that, as a teenager, I had periods of being blue, feeling that I had no friends, feeling that life was hopeless. They were trying times because of the Vietnam War. I had trouble walking around, and nightmares. It wasn't just a minor thing. If I had to put a date on it I would say probably the mid-sixties.

Then I started getting over-excited — I think it was probably when I was at university. At the time I just enjoyed it — it didn't register that I was not sleeping for days and getting garrulous, or that my friends were becoming impatient with me. I was physically overactive, too. Sometimes this would occur after I'd been feeling down for long periods. It was such a relief to experience the other side of things that I never considered it a problem. In fact I wished it would happen more often, but it didn't. I got depressed more often.

I went to student counsellors for some assistance when I was at university. They were trained psychologists. I now look back with very disillusioned feelings. From one woman I used to get anger: 'Why don't you interest yourself in other people more? Why don't you try this? Why don't you do that?' It was always my fault that I was feeling depressed. I went to another fellow, and he was a bit more understanding about it, but nothing was ever mentioned about treatment. It was all situational things: 'Why don't you go up into the bush, why don't you go to see a film or something, and alter the environment a bit and you'll feel better?' So I didn't get any help with depression, and I never sought help for being over-excited because that didn't worry me. Even now I miss not feeling it.

When I came to Australia I experienced depression... That was after my father died. I was in hospital anyway. I had an operation, and then I got glandular fever. Then I became very depressed, and people said it was because my father had died, which may have been true, but I don't think so now. The doctor prescribed antidepressants. 'Take these and you'll be better in a week or two.' I was not better in a week and I stopped taking them.

I got depressed again and it was always this stop-gap business. One time I just couldn't stop crying. I went to see the doctor, and I remember being annoyed because I was talking and he was writing some prescription and ignoring me. I understand why: he knew what was wrong. He finally said, 'Why don't you go and see a psychiatrist, because I really can't help you.' I did, and it was only then that it was explained to me what was wrong, and that there were drugs that could be useful. I used some for a short time and then things seemed to be okay. I didn't get depressed again for quite a while. Then, about six years ago, things began to get very depressing and I had very long depressions with very deep suicidal undertones. I couldn't manage those at all.

I was simply obsessed with the fact that I needed to die. The problems I was experiencing were insoluble, and were centred on me, with my own inadequacy, my own blunderings. Therefore if I eliminated myself I would eliminate the problem. I felt that I could not escape. Those thoughts were relentless, so I spent a lot of time planning what I was going to do to myself.

I tried to commit suicide. I would have been dead, except that Susie found me. I have no recollection of what I did; I just woke up in a hospital a few days later. The drive to kill myself had been overwhelming. I remember being angry when I awoke: how dare people interfere! I was furious, because then I was back where I'd been before.

I've had two kinds of elation. One kind is when I'm simply in fast speed, I'm moving more quickly, I'm talking more quickly, my ideas flip from one thing to the next. I'm full of enthusiasm for whatever happens to be at hand at the moment, which of course can change quickly to something else. I become insensitive to other people's moods, and other people in general. But, then there was another kind where I couldn't think at all, where everything was going just too quickly. I couldn't drive because of how fast I was going. When the traffic lights were about to change, it was a very difficult thing to work out when to put the foot on the brake. Changing lanes was just too complicated, and watching for other people, so I stopped driving.

My psychiatrist said not to carry any money when I was elated so that I wouldn't have any to spend, and not to go shopping when I was depressed because I'd be likely to shoplift. I had people around me, so I wasn't left to my own devices for too long. I never did anything that I was sorry about. Some people get entirely carried away, but I never got that far. What I tend to do is go dancing, and I'll just dance all night, then rage all day and then go dancing the next night. I like to go out for nights on end when I am high. I get into lots of laughter: things appear to be funny that I suppose are only mildly humorous. People get sick of it, they don't like it and they run out of ways to cope with it. They become detached. The only way they can cope with it, I suppose, is not to get emotionally involved, because it isn't real. So it causes a great deal of tension in the home.

At first my psychiatrist wanted to work out how depressed I was, so he used antidepressants very sparingly. He asked me to keep records of how I was going. It became apparent soon that the bouts were going on for lengthy periods and they weren't going away. So I tried a variety of tricyclics over a couple of years. None of them really worked. They would work to the point of controlling some of the negative thoughts I was having all the time.

Being depressed for me is being very negative about myself. It's being hopeless, blaming, feeling guilty, and being full of delusions. I get fears that aren't real and I know they're not real... When I'm depressed I develop the fear that I'm an alcoholic and that I've got a real problem because of it. And yet when I'm not depressed, like now, I don't drink very much. It's apparent that I'm not an alcoholic, but I know that, if I'm depressed, that will become not just a passing fear, it will keep me awake at night. It doesn't matter what reality shows us, that's how it feels.

I also imagine that I don't have any friends at all. That is a very frightening experience. Never mind that there are people sitting next to me. I'll spend a long time telling people that I'm lonely, that no one loves me, and I'm unlovable, and all those negative things. It's apparent that if people didn't care they wouldn't be there. I get fears of illness or impending doom. I get one pain and I think I'm having a heart attack, or I get another pain and something else is wrong. Even though the doctor tells me there's nothing, the fears don't go away. I guess the greatest fear of all is that of losing my sanity. Not ever being on top of things again, never just being normal, never thinking straight and being able to study again.

When I'm depressed I have trouble moving. If I have trouble pedalling when I'm riding my bicycle, that is a clear indication to me that the depression is beginning to reach a low level. I ride all the time, and sometimes when I tried to ride to work it was just so hard, and I was so tired, that my legs would hurt. It would take me twice as long to get there.

I think the children have accepted sometimes that I don't get out of bed, because I'm crying or unhappy. They'll come in and try to cheer me up. I think with Susie it just causes a distance. It's beginning to get better now, but I think for a couple of years, when nothing seemed to be helping, she figured what's the point of maintaining a relationship with someone who is obviously not much fun to be around, and who's always destructive. Not on purpose, but that tends to be the impact of it. 'Let's go out to a party,' she'll say, and I'll be enthusiastic. Then it's time to go and I'm too depressed, and I don't want to see anybody. It's happened: we were going to go to a party and I started crying before we left the house.

It's hard to share your feelings with someone who is unable to appreciate them. My psychiatrist suggested that it could take several years for that gulf to be healed. He said in any mental illness, it doesn't matter what it is, you can cure the individual but the family has to catch up later. It takes them longer. Even when you are feeling better they don't trust you.

I went on lithium several years ago. When I was going through a changeover from one kind of tricyclic to another, I got really high. Absolutely higher than I'd ever experienced before. So, I went right back to the psychiatrist and said something was wrong. He said it could be that the swings were getting worse, or it could be a one-off thing. He said I could try lithium, but must understand that it would be a long-term thing. You can't take it and then stop taking it. He explained the side-effects. It was my choice what to do, so I tried it.

As a result of lithium treatment I experienced the greatest peace of mind I have ever known in my whole life. Couldn't stop talking about the relief. I wrote to my mother and explained it to her. I said I had just come to understand that I was having more swings than I was conscious of. Then I stopped taking lithium to see whether I would still get high again, and I did, so it was decided that I would continue taking it. I now enjoy peace of mind, I enjoy the freedom from those swings, and I have a great deal of pride. I'm proud of the fact that no one can tell that I used to be a problem. Some people have commented on how even-tempered I am. I haven't told anyone, but people have noticed it. They say, 'Gee, you seem to be happier these days, or things are a bit calmer. You don't worry about things as you used to.'

I do enjoy the experience of getting high — I can't say that I don't. I have stopped taking it occasionally just to regain that experience but I can also tell when things are getting out of hand and it's time to start up again. The last time I stopped taking it was a coincidence. I was going to a dance. I had a great time but by the following afternoon I told myself this was not normal, not right for me. Since then I've decided not to do that.

The difference is that now, when I'm feeling blue, I still have resilience. Somebody can crack a joke and I'll still laugh. I might be feeling a bit lethargic and a bit low... but I can still enjoy good food or people. I can do that. Whereas without the drugs it's just a relentless down feeling.

My psychiatrist offers several services. One is that he looks after my physical health, and then the second thing is that sometimes crises arise in life that he can help me cope with. Thirdly, he is a person who understands my illness, and if I'm puzzled or not feeling well, I can go to him. I have a sense of trust that he is able to help me. Also he's a very... nice, warm person. Sometimes I go to see him and there is really nothing to talk about. I get my prescriptions filled in and then I see him in a few months, and at other times I can ring him up right away and say, 'I'm feeling bad about something and I can't handle it, can I come and see you?' And he'll make time to see me. I'm never prodded and I'm never pushed; I'm never hurt. Suggestions are made which I can follow up if I wish and don't have to if I don't want to. It's been very beneficial and I know that I've grown from the experience.

I started psychology studies before I was having trouble at the school. I decided that I wanted to be something different; perhaps it was just because of my age. Psychology had interested me, because I'd done it as an undergraduate, and I knew that my knowledge was out of date. I guess what I want to do now is finish the course. I want to work in a new job with adults. I don't want to work with children any more, and I need that competition and sense of meaning. I'm sick to death of facing antagonism, sick of it, and it's not good for my mental health, I know that. I've learnt a lot through this experience, and I'm just going to finish the psychology course and do some practical experience. Then I'll wait and see what jobs come along.

At the moment I'm really dedicated to my kids. I love being home with them, and I really enjoy being with Susie.

I do lots of volunteer work with two other groups in the city, so that takes up a bit of my time. I've joined a telephone counselling group and I work with adults weekly, sometimes every other week. It depends on the needs of the service at the time. Sometimes in the day, sometimes at night. I work with people who have AIDS and need different types of assistance, and that's rewarding. Just all the forces involved in that, including all the training I've had to go through to learn how to deal with sufferers, has made me grow enormously. I guess it is a bit of a positive thing for me. I know that, despite my own troubles, I've been doing that very successfully. That's why I don't have any doubts at all about my new study of psychology. I'm proving to myself that the troubles that I've had don't really matter. It is a little bit like the problem is contained. It's a bit like I had a broken leg and now it's healed. I can carry people up stairs if I need to.

MANAGEMENT AND TREATMENT STRATEGIES

There is a stigma attached to any disorder of the mind, although with increasing education and publicity the stigma is lessening. It is still, overall, a social handicap if you are being treated by a psychiatrist. It is even more difficult if the disorder from which you suffer has resulted in socially unacceptable, embarrassing, maritally disruptive or financially ruinous behaviour, as occurs in mania, or has resulted in attempted suicide, as happens in severe depression only too often.

Terminology has played a key role in hindering progress towards the removal of such a stigma. For many people, the term 'manic-depressive psychosis' is reminiscent of a whole range of tags — among them 'psycho', 'loony', 'schizo', 'maniac', 'spastic' and 'imbecile' — which originally derive from accurate terminology used by the medical profession, but have come to be traded as insults in street and domestic arguments.

Patients and psychiatrists alike now seem to prefer the term *bipolar mood disorder.* If it comes into general usage, it is certainly unlikely to descend into the realms of insult — 'You're a bipolar mood disorder!' is never going to be as catchy or provocative as 'You're a maniac' or 'She's manic-depressive'.

It is hoped that the conquering of this first hurdle in the process of gradual enlightenment will equip more people to understand the issues involved in managing and treating bipolar mood disorder.

Mania and major depression are medical crises. While most psychiatrists would agree that the management of these disorders is stressful and demanding, they would also agree that it is one of the most rewarding aspects of being a psychiatrist. If the problem is managed well there is nearly always a successful outcome, and the outlook for mood disorder is probably better than for any other serious disorder that psychiatrists treat.

Support

People with bipolar mood disorder are usually members of a family unit or at least a social community. This means that they have a support network which offers not only crucial encouragement, understanding and mechanisms for rebuilding self-esteem but also practical management of the problem.

Such a support network has an important role to play in the recognition of early warning signs. Because of the very nature of their illness, patients are often unable to do this alone.

Professor W A Cramond, a Scottish-born psychiatrist who has made a major contribution to Australian psychiatry, has emphasised the value of having a plan based on recognising early warning signs of mania and major depression in order to prevent a full-blown relapse. Professor Cramond was the founding patron of Mood Disturbance Prevention (Inc.), or MDP, a very successful self-help group based at Glenside Hospital in Adelaide but serving the whole of South Australia.

The experience of MDP is that, once the sufferer and their carer have been well educated about mood disorder, especially after a bout of illness, together they can compile a list of at least six early warning signs, which are almost always the same for any one person.

Working with their therapist, the patient can develop an action plan which can be used even if the therapist is not immediately available. For example, two-thirds of the maximum medication ever prescribed for the patient can quite safely be taken for one week, followed by half of the maximum for a further week, after which consultation with the therapist should again be possible.

Early warning signs can be used as an effective management tool to produce a cycle of: stressors — early warning signs — appropriate action — control — wellness and so on, instead of allowing hospitalisation to become an inevitability.

In some cases the support network itself might need some assistance in coping with the trauma of mood disorder. Young people, in particular, have difficulty in accepting that biological illness can cause psychiatric symptoms, among them unprecedented hostility from a parent developing mania. In their youthful zeal and their ignorance of medical facts, they are likely to urge a depressed parent to just 'snap out of it'.

On top of their confusion they are usually faced with the difficult role adjustment of being expected to take on parental responsibilities. Further difficulties can arise after the recovery of the patient, when young family members who have assumed adult roles are then expected to go back to doing what they are told by the recovered parent.

Family conferences which include the depressed or hypomanic patient often help to clarify attitudes and feelings produced by these problems, making way for much-needed family support for the ill member. Someone suffering major depression has feelings of guilt and poor self-esteem, and can well do without rejection from those closest to them.

Meetings involving the family, the patient and the psychiatrist are also useful in clarifying family concerns about treatment, particularly medication, and (above all) electroconvulsive therapy. If relatives are on side with the psychiatrist and the rest of the treatment team, they can often help to persuade depressed patients who believe that treatment is useless, or hypomanic patients who believe that it is unnecessary, to take the prescribed treatment.

If the hospital has a psychiatric social worker on its staff the knowledge and skills of such a professional can be put to good use in working with the family. Some people are more comfortable with a social worker than a psychiatrist because they feel intimidated by the perceived status of the medical profession, though nowadays less commonly than in the past.

Self-help

As a result of the relatively recent movement which encourages people to become responsible for maintaining their own health and manage their ailments, self-help groups for sufferers of many physical and psychiatric disorders have developed around the world.

Groups for those who suffer mood swings can be found throughout Australia. Mood Disturbance Prevention (Inc.), which has already been mentioned, was founded in 1983 and can lay claim to being the first body in Australia to develop an organised programme and network for large numbers of people with mood disorder.

Under the leadership of founder and Executive Director

Richard Woon, himself a sufferer, and strongly supported by psychiatrists and other health care professionals, it has encouraged the formation of groups in other States and New Zealand, and has been used as a model by many of them.

MDP's philosophy is based on long experience and emphasises the importance of educating carers as well as patients, not only in recognising early warning signs but also in sharing experiences in a constructive way and, above all, in taking primary responsibility for one's own illness and how it is treated.

Not everybody finds self-help groups of benefit, for various reasons which include a desire for anonymity, and personality factors. On the other hand they greatly improve many people's ability to cope and to enjoy life in spite of the presence of bipolar disorder.

The addresses and telephone numbers of known groups in various States and in New Zealand, and Mental Health Foundations, which may know of other groups, are listed in Appendix V.

Hospitalisation and Outpatient Treatment

For people suffering from mania or suicidal depression, the risks associated with being left out in the community, and the intensity of the treatment required, make the management decision easy: there is no practical alternative to hospital admission. On the other hand, a person with mild depression or the lesser degrees of hypomania can, with adequate family or social supports, be safely managed as an outpatient. The problem is that the severity of this disorder, in both its manic and depressed phases, is on a sliding scale, and it is the management of the grey area between the mild and the very severe that requires experience, skill and judgement.

To declare that the severely ill must be admitted to hospital is easy; to get them there is not. Manic patients rarely retain sufficient insight to recognise the extent of their illness and may need certifying, or sometimes just the threat of certification, to effect admission.

Often the situation is taken out of the doctor's hands, as the person with mania may, by their unlawful or antisocial behaviour, attract the attention of the police. The latter are usually sufficiently experienced to recognise mania for what it is, and too busy to spend the time required to persuade the person to accept voluntary admission. The usual result is that the person is certified and admitted as an involuntary patient.

If a patient is given the option between certification and voluntary admission they will usually choose the latter, provided that the most significant people in their life decide clearly in their own minds that hospitalisation is essential. If they tell the patient that it is, but in their hearts could not stand to see the patient certified (even if that is the only way to get them into hospital), the patient senses their reluctance and, paradoxically, usually finishes up being certified. If the relatives or friends decide that hospitalisation is the only option, the psychotic patient, who is usually very sensitive to covert messages, will 'get the message' and agree to voluntary admission.

Skilled nursing is essential in the management of patients in the psychotic stage of mood disorder. They need close supervision to ensure that they receive adequate fluid and food intake, close attention to personal hygiene, and the professional degree of reassurance and support that psychiatric nurses are trained to give.

A patient requiring intensive psychiatric care might be difficult to control. Whereas in authorised hospitals the patient might be confined to a locked ward, in most private hospitals they must be managed, by law, in an unlocked ward, and this requires a high staff presence. Private hospitals are now developing intensive psychiatric care units, with much higher staff ratios than in general wards, as pioneered in Australia by The Melbourne Clinic. This has meant that many privately insured patients, who would formerly have had to be transferred to public hospitals with the right to lock patients in, can now be treated without the humiliation of certification.

On the other hand, the psychotically depressed might have difficulty in agreeing to hospitalisation because of their belief that they are doomed and so treatment is useless. The matter is complicated if there is also a delusion of poverty.

The patient with major depressive illness who is suicidal, who has given up hope and therefore will not co-operate with treatment at home, or has become severely wasted and sometimes dehydrated, obviously requires hospitalisation. Other reasons for admission are personal or business circumstances which impose a time limit on a sufferer's restoration to health.

Any patient whose condition deteriorates while they are being treated as an outpatient, or fails to improve after reasonable time, also warrants admission. Some patients are so weak that they need to be nursed in bed and spoon fed. On occasions a patient who has been living alone, or neglected by uncaring members of the family, will need intravenous infusions to restore body fluids to safe levels.

For the less severely mentally ill many factors will be involved in a decision as to where to treat the sufferer. In the public sector, in particular, there is a movement towards managing the psychiatrically ill within the community, using community-based treatment teams. In the private sector there is no funding available for such community-based treatment, and the resources of a hospital are more often needed. However, better education of medical students has enabled family doctors, physicians and even surgeons to recognise psychiatric illness earlier, and thus to treat or refer the patient earlier and minimise the need for hospital admission. As well as the degree of impairment caused by the illness, the effect on the family, the family resources, and (for those living outside the major centres of population) geographical factors must all be considered in assessing the need for admission.

Hospitalisation of psychiatric patients has an important benefit that is not always understood. Unlike other hospitals, where patients are confined to bed, the regimen in a psychiatric hospital combines professional treatment with the encouragement of a daily routine that simulates the life of someone living in the community.

Except in the initial or acute stages, when rest might be one of the main priorities, patients are required to get out of bed at a reasonable hour, shower, dress and have breakfast, in readiness for a programme of daily activities. This deters them from lying in bed all morning, missing meals and becoming socially withdrawn — behaviour that commonly persists amongst those who are not hospitalised.

At a first class psychiatric hospital activities are provided for patients, no matter what their level of functioning. Manual and creative pursuits, group discussions, social skills training, relaxation and stress management, music, and gardening interests are some of the activities provided in daily programmes organised by the nursing and occupational therapy departments.

The overall aim is to maintain or upgrade functioning in all areas required for daily living.

Treatment as an Integrated Whole

Any one patient might be treated with a combination of medications and therapies. These are not mutually exclusive; patients taking medication will also frequently see their therapist, who will encourage them to continue with medication even if there is an apparent lack of progress, discuss the way they are feeling, and explore the origins of their problem and strategies that might lead to recovery.

Some patients in cognitive therapy or dynamic psychotherapy will not be on medications, but most will. When a patient is hospitalised, nurses and occupational therapists, and social workers in many instances, will also be responsible for their care and treatment.

Good therapists combine a range of available therapies in treating a patient, and often call upon the skills of colleagues specialising in one mode of therapy or another.

Medications

A number of medications are used to treat mood disorder. Some are effective only for mania, others only for severe depression; and many are effective for both.

It is not an exaggeration to say that drugs developed in the last thirty years have revolutionised the treatment of mania in particular. In countries that can (or do) afford the use of these drugs, the straitjacket has disappeared and the once-common scene of a manic patient confined to a cage is now just a tragic part of psychiatric history.

In the initial stages the most common drugs used to bring a manic episode under control are the phenothiazine drugs haloperidol (Serenace®) and chlorpromazine (Largactil®). Often very large doses are given, at frequent intervals and with close observation to avoid overdosage. As these drugs take effect the dosage is rapidly reduced. A longer-term treatment, lithium carbonate, is usually commenced at the same time, as it takes one or two weeks to be effective.

The drugs used to treat mania (as with all drugs used in medicine), have side-effects. They all cause dryness of the mouth, constipation and, in the doses used, blurring of vision, stiffness of the muscles and tremor. The latter two symptoms are part of the syndrome known as Parkinsonism but they respond to other drugs and disappear when the anti-manic drug is ceased.

Chlorpromazine (Largactil®) is the more sedative of the two drugs most often used. In addition to calming the manic over-activity, it produces sleepiness, often to an undesirable degree. It also causes low blood pressure which can result in patients falling when they stand up. Haloperidol (Serenace®) does not produce as much lowering of blood pressure, but is likely to produce more severe side-effects of the Parkinsonian type (stiffness of the limbs, tremor, restlessness, and so on).

These drugs, especially when combined with lithium, might (rarely) cause a severe reaction (stupor, abnormal movements and a high temperature), which can be fatal. Psychiatrists continue to use them because this complication is rare, can usually be treated successfully and the alternative (not using drugs for treatment) might in any case result in the patient's death from manic excitement and exhaustion.

Tricyclic Antidepressants (TCAs)

It is rare for a person in the depressed phase of bipolar mood disorder to respond to treatment that does not include medication or electroconvulsive therapy. For most patients the treatment of first choice is an antidepressant, particularly the group known as tricyclic antidepressants (so named because they contain three rings of atoms in their chemical structure), which have been used for over thirty years. No particular member of this group has been shown to be more effective than the others, and the drug which is the personal preference of the psychiatrist is likely to be prescribed.

Although they are likely to be equally effective overall, individuals do vary and the choice will be influenced if a patient has responded to one particular drug in the past, or if a close member of the family has responded well to a certain drug.

Tricyclic antidepressants (TCAs) do not act as a stimulant, as does, for example, amphetamine ('speed'). They might not be fully effective for many weeks, though most patients start to feel the benefit in the second week of therapy. In bipolar patients they can cause a shift into hypomania, which requires rapid adjustment of the dosage, and either an increase in the dosage of lithium if the patient is already taking that drug, or commencement of lithium therapy.

Side-effects from TCAs are common and often troublesome; though, as in the drugs used for the treatment of mania, the benefits justify encouraging the patients to tolerate the side-effects so that they can obtain relief from their painful illness. Common side-effects are tiredness, dryness of the mouth, constipation, blurring of vision, tremor and low blood pressure resulting in the tendency to faint. Some of the new drugs, such as dothiepin and mianserin, have fewer side-effects, though they do produce sedation. As a rule, side-effects decrease with time. For this reason the starting dose is usually well below the dose needed to produce an effective response in the patient and it is gradually increased as the patient becomes accustomed to the drug.

The concentration of the drug in the body for any given dose varies greatly between individuals, and the eventual daily dose will depend upon the patient's response and the severity of side-effects. The blurring of vision is largely limited to close work, and is distressing for both manic and depressed patients, who are often unable to read because of it. Inexpensive glasses of varying strengths can be obtained over the counter to correct this problem and are a boon to many patients.

One side-effect often complained about is excessive weight gain, which is partly due to an increased appetite for sweet foods but is probably also an effect of the medication on the metabolism.

The Melbourne Clinic has prepared a guide to TCAs detailing side-effects and their management as well as general information on the action of this group of drugs (see Appendix IV).

Monoamine Oxidase Inhibitors (MAOIs)

Monoamine oxidase inhibitors, commonly referred to as MAOIs, are another group of drugs used in the treatment of major depression. They are rarely the first choice in treating the disorder because of the dietary and other restrictions that patients must follow when taking them.

These restrictions are necessary because the MAOIs can interact with other ingested substances to produce a sudden and severe rise in blood pressure which causes a very severe headache and can result in a fatal stroke. Foods containing tyramine, particularly matured cheeses and meat extracts (Vegemite®, Marmite®, Bonox®) must be avoided. There are many other banned foods, most of which are not part of a basic diet (as cheese usually is), and a number of medications, including non-prescription cough and cold remedies, that must also be avoided.

The restrictions and dangers would, on the face of it, seem a good reason not to use this group of drugs, which include phenelzine (Nardil®), tranylcypromine (Parnate®) and tranylcypromine with trifluoperazine (Parstelin®). However, to put the risks in perspective, severe reactions are rare. Many high-blood-pressure reactions have resulted from wrong advice given by family doctors and pharmacists, so it is sound practice to advise patients taking MAOIs to check with their psychiatrist or a drug information centre before taking a new medication.

There are effective antidotes which will rapidly reduce the blood pressure to normal — one of which, chlorpromazine, would be found in most family doctors' surgeries.

There are many lists available of the foods and drugs to be avoided when MAOIs are being taken. Some are not comprehensive enough; others too restrictive (they include foods with a minimal, non-dangerous, amount of tyramine). The Melbourne Clinic has prepared a guide for patients which has been approved by the Victorian Health Department Office of Psychiatric Services Drug Information Centre and is included in this book as Appendix III.

MAOIs have other side-effects that are similar to those of tricyclic antidepressants — dry mouth, constipation, low blood pressure on standing, and weight gain. Nevertheless, they sometimes prove effective when tricyclic antidepressants have failed. At times their beneficial effect can be much enhanced when combined with lithium (this can also occur when lithium is added to tricyclic antidepressants).

Lithium

The benefits of lithium in the treatment of mania were discovered by Dr John Cade, a Melbourne psychiatrist, who first published a paper on his treatment in the *Medical Journal of Australia* in 1949. Before 1949, the best that could be done for a person suffering from mania was physical restraint and the use of relatively ineffective and dangerous sedative drugs, though at times electroconvulsive therapy terminated an episode. The manic phase might continue for weeks, months or even years. For major depression the picture improved with the introduction of electroconvulsive therapy in the 1930s. However, nothing could be done to prevent recurrence of bipolar mood disorder until the advent of lithium as a treatment.

Dr John Cade first established its beneficial effect on a manic episode, though as is so often the case, history provided a precedent. The ancient-Greek physicians recommended that sufferers from over-elation should drink the waters of certain spas, which still exist today and have been found to contain high levels of lithium.

It took some time for the treatment to be accepted because the dose required to produce an effective response was so close to being toxic. It was taken up by a Danish psychiatrist, Dr Mogens Schou and he and others discovered in the early 1950s that it not only terminated the episode of mania but, if given continuously, largely prevented recurrences of both mania and depression. This work, combined with the development of relatively simple and accurate ways of measuring the level of lithium in the blood, has led to the universal use of lithium to treat bipolar mood disorder.

Dr Cade, who died in 1981, received international honours for his discovery, though sadly did not receive adequate recognition from his own country. An Australian psychiatrist had a moving experience when a Chinese psychiatrist in the far west of that country asked whether he could touch him, simply because he had been taught by Dr John Cade.

The United States of America, whose Food and Drug Administration (FDA) are notoriously severe in assessing drugs for approval, took more than twenty years to recognise the unique value of lithium as a treatment for mood disorder. The delay was partly due to deaths from lithium toxicity when it was used as a substitute for common salt in patients with heart failure in the 1940s, before practicable methods of measuring serum lithium levels were developed. (Even today, the US FDA does not approve of its use as a treatment for unipolar depression.) But it could also be due to the fact that lithium is an abundant natural substance not subject to patent and with little profitability for those who market it. This at least makes it economically viable for use in the Third World.

Psychiatrists have found that, in about ninety per cent of patients, the continuous taking of lithium will prevent episodes of illness severe enough to warrant hospitalisation, and in seventy-five per cent of patients it will eliminate significant episodes of mood swings altogether. However, it is one thing for psychiatrists to be aware of these benefits; it is entirely another for patients to accept that, on a cost- benefit analysis, lithium therapy is worthwhile to prevent recurrence. People are, by nature, optimists (some have suggested if the population consisted entirely of realists, mass suicide would be the order of the day); if they have one attack of illness they believe it will never happen again, and some people who have many attacks still cling to the belief that each one will be their last.

Influential family members may be against medication, particularly the idealistic young. For some people the mere thought of having regular blood tests is a strong disincentive to taking lithium. Psychiatrists would agree that, on the debit side, in addition to the problems associated with accepting that one has a chronic illness, and the need for blood tests, lithium has significant side-effects. These include, in the early stages, nausea, tremor and thirst. Nausea usually eases, but a mild tremor, thirst and passing more urine often persist. Another common side-effect is weight gain; while lethargy, skin changes and low thyroid function are rarer problems.

However, having seen the devastation in the personal and wider world of patients suffering from this disorder, and knowing the risk of death through suicide or accident, most psychiatrists agree that a person who has suffered two or three episodes of mood disorder (including episodes of mania sufficiently severe to warrant hospitalisation) in as many years, should have a trial of lithium therapy.

The side-effects, and the more serious toxic effects of lithium, are discussed in more detail in Appendix II, which is a modified version of a brochure available from The Melbourne Clinic. Many psychiatrists in private and public practice have copies for distribution to patients, their relatives and doctors.

Other Medications

Some patients respond neither to the standard medications (TCAs and MAOIs) nor to ECT; that is, they have what is called treatment-resistant depression.

For these patients, less commonly prescribed treatments are necessary. Psychiatrists will differ about the order in which the other treatments should be tried.

Tryptophan, an amino acid found in the normal diet, was once sometimes added to the medication regime in fairly large quantities (up to four grams a day) but is now suspected of occasionally causing very serious side-effects and is no longer used. The addition of thyroxine (a hormone produced by the thyroid gland) has been known to be effective.

One of the more controversial medication regimes is the combination of TCAs and MAOIs. Many authorities regard the mixtures as dangerous, yet leaders in the treatment of mood disorder, such as Dr William Sargant of England and Dr Frank Ayd Jnr. of the USA, have used it safely and effectively as a treatment for a large number of patients over many years. The extreme gratitude of patients when it works is understandable, as they are likely to have spent many months of despair trying more orthodox treatments.

New antidepressants are coming onto the market at frequent intervals. Some turn out to be relatively ineffective, and some have adverse side-effects. The most successful in recent times is fluoxetine (Prozac 20®), which is about as effective as tricyclic antidepressants and does not have some of their side-effects (dry mouth, blurred vision, constipation, palpitations, sweating, weight gain). It can have its own side-effects (headache, nausea, insomnia, nervousness, sleepiness) but most people tolerate it well.

Another medication approved for use in Australian in 1992 is moclobemide (Aurorix®), which is an MAOI but has important differences from the MAOIs already mentioned. As a result, the food and drug restrictions placed upon this medication are not nearly so stringent.

For patients in whom lithium is not effective or for whom the side-effects are intolerable, the most commonly used alternative is carbamazepine (Tegretol®), which is primarily an anti-epileptic medication but is used in some other disorders of the nervous system. Clonazepan (Rivotril®) is a benzodiazepine (Valium®-type) drug which is also primarily an anti-convulsant, but often used in the acute treatment of a manic episode and sometimes as a long-term treatment. Another anti-convulsant, sodium valproate (Epilim®) has sometimes been found to be useful when other medications don't suit the patient.

Agitation and anxiety, although less common in the depressed phase of bipolar disorder than in unipolar disorder, might require benzodiazepines or one of the phenothiazine group of drugs (such as those used in the treatment of mania). (See page 65.)

Electroconvulsive Therapy (ECT)

Studies suggest that electroconvulsive therapy ('shock therapy' or ECT) is more effective than medication in the treatment of severe depression. However, the unwarranted horror with which many, perhaps a majority, in the community, react to the proposed use of this treatment means that it is usually reserved for cases in which drugs fail or are contraindicated.

The evidence is that ECT is safe, is more likely to be effective than medication and more rapid in producing remission, is relatively free of side-effects in both the short and the long term, is cost-effective and has the added benefit that the patient cannot overdose on it.

In forming the lay public's impression of ECT, nothing has been as powerful as the book (and subsequent film) *One Flew Over The Cuckoo's Nest,* which is regularly on the English syllabus in the final two years of secondary education in Australia.

It is quite common for people who read the story or viewed the film to believe that the terrible treatments depicted in the story, including ECT, are an accurate picture of treatment in psychiatric hospitals. Indeed, an architect appointed to design the ECT suite of The Melbourne Clinic asked about the amount of sound insulation needed to muffle the screams. When told repeatedly that there were no screams, he countered by saying, 'I know what goes on — I saw *One Flew Over The Cuckoo's Nest*'. Assurances that the film was not a documentary but a fictional work were to no avail. When the constructed suite was inspected it was discovered that the wall between it and the outside corridor was full of lead!

Because of the unwarranted notoriety surrounding ECT, which results in patients and relatives tending to throw up their hands in horror at the suggestion that it should be given, it is usually a second choice treatment. However, in the actively suicidal patient, those with delusions and those who have physical wasting and are sometimes almost comatose as a result of their depressive illness, it is the psychiatrist's first choice of treatment.

Legislation provides that ECT cannot be given without what is known as written informed consent, as is required for any operation and many medical procedures. However, only in the case of ECT and operations on the brain for psychiatric disorders does the law in Australia lay down the extent of information required to be given.

It is so extremely complex — including requirements to name all alternative treatments and every possible risk of the procedure, and to inform the patient that they have the right to have a lawyer advise them about signing consent — that, if the same rules were applied to all medical procedures (and that may yet come), few people would allow their children to be immunised, let alone submit themselves to any surgical operation.

The media have some responsibility for the anti-ECT propaganda which has influenced governments to put such unprecedented restrictions on the use of a safe, effective, and at times life-saving treatment. Some individuals and organisations are anti-medical and, in particular, anti-psychiatry, and make very dubious claims about ECT causing significant, even severe, brain damage. They receive frequent exposure in the press without producing any scientifically acceptable evidence of dangers to human beings from the treatment.

However, it is not only the so-called 'lunatic fringe' that opposes ECT. Some well-meaning social workers and other health professionsls in positions to influence health policy and delivery often have an anti-medical, anti-psychiatrist attitude; and governments, while riddled with lawyers, tend to contain very few medical practitioners. There are certainly very few psychiatrists in positions of real authority in health departments in Australia.

In this setting it was not altogether surprising when an official hospital visitor, with responsibility for seeing that patients in State hospitals get proper treatment, recently protested that patients who were suffering from a type of depression necessitating ECT treatment were being certified because they were not willing or able to give informed consent.

Psychiatrists who put forward rational arguments about ECT are often accused of having a vested interest in the procedure. Jerome L Gelb, a young Melbourne psychiatrist, responded to one such accusation in Melbourne's *Age* newspaper with the following cogent letter:

'The appointment of community visitors under the Mental Health Act, Victoria, (1986) had the potential not only to provide for greater public scrutiny of mental health service delivery, but to diminish the fear and ignorance of mental illness and its treatment that leads to continued stigmatisation of our patients.

'The letter by W Jordan, community visitor is therefore

terribly disappointing. Despite ample evidence in the literature to the contrary, Mr Jordan perpetuates the mythology promulgated by anti-psychiatry groups throughout Australia. It is obvious that he has neither studied the available evidence, nor observed the therapeutic use of ECT in Victoria.

'The interests of psychiatrists are indeed vested; vested in their patients' recovery of good health. May I inform your readers that untreated depressive illness has a mortality rate of 15 per cent, that not all patients respond to medication or psychotherapy, and that ECT is an effective, safe treatment with a mortality rate equivalent to that of a dental procedure done under general anaesthesia (three per 100,000 treatments).'

A patient who had received ECT and who was brave enough to ignore the stigma associated with it (a stigma which has resulted in one US presidential candidate being forced to withdraw) also wrote a letter to the *Age* in response to the same attack on ECT:

'As someone who has been treated with ECT, I would like to add to comments already made in the Age regarding electro-convulsive therapy (ECT).

'I first received ECT as treatment for chronically severe depression after I failed to respond to a number of other treatments, including antidepressant medication and psychotherapy.

'It was given only after careful consideration and after I fully understood what it involved.

'Initially I was fearful and apprehensive at the prospect of having ECT and thought it would stigmatise me as mentally inferior. I soon realised otherwise: I was genuinely sick, in need of help and this was the best form of treatment available for me.

'It gave me periods of relief from the debilitating nature of my illness and prevented me acting upon the suicidal thoughts which plagued me. It also gave me the much-needed hope that something positive could be done as well as enabling me to benefit from other forms of treatment.

'Certainly there are side-effects and risks associated with ECT but, with competent administration by a skilled specialist and careful supervision, these can be minimised. In fact, there are side-effects and risks associated with most forms of treatment and, of greater concern, with depression itself.

'In the final analysis the wellbeing of the patient becomes

the primary consideration and, if indicated, ECT should be offered as a valuable and respectable form of treatment. I am grateful for the part it played in my own recovery and would undergo it again if circumstances warranted it.'

Let us look at this controversial procedure — its history, development and how it is administered.

Convulsive therapy, using injections of camphor, was first given in 1934 by a Viennese psychiatrist, L J von Meduna, at a time when Freudian psychoanalytical theories held sway and physical treatments were eschewed.

The basis for the use of this treatment was the belief that epilepsy and schizophrenia were antagonistic and rarely occurred together. This hypothesis was soon called into question, but the psychiatrists using convulsive therapy observed that, though it was not very successful in treating schizophrenia, it was very effective in the treatment of mood disorders, especially severe depression.

In 1938 two Italians, Cerletti and Bini, developed a method of inducing convulsions by applying an electric current to the scalp. This had many advantages over chemical means of inducing fits, and so was a major contribution to the treatment of suffering patients. In retrospect they probably rued giving the treatment the name 'electro shock', as the term has fuelled the fire of controversy. The facts are that patients do not feel a shock, nor do they suffer from shock — as, say, after excessive bleeding.

In the fifty or so years since the work of Cerletti and Bini the equipment used has been steadily improved so that the amount of current required to produce a convulsion has been markedly reduced.

One of the most important advances has been the introduction of intravenous muscle relaxants, such as are used in most major surgical operations. Because the muscle-relaxing drugs paralyse breathing, and if the patient is conscious this produces a feeling of suffocation, it is preceded by a short-acting intravenous anaesthetic such as thiopentone (the usual way of putting a patient to sleep before an operation). The muscle relaxant enables the convulsion to proceed in the brain without the violent muscle contractions that occur in a spontaneous fit. This prevents damage to muscles and sinews.

The anaesthetist administers oxygen through a face mask

and an oxygen bag and once the signs of muscle relaxation are detected in the now-unconscious patient, the psychiatrist supplies two electrodes to the scalp, either one on each temple or two on one side — nearly always the right-hand side. (Psychiatric opinion differs on which is the best — bilateral or unilateral application, but the difference is minor and difficult to determine.)

A current of about one ampere travels through the brain and induces the modified convulsion which lasts for up to a minute. At the conclusion the patient is again given oxygen until the effect of the muscle relaxant wears off and normal breathing returns, which usually takes a minute or so.

The patient is turned on the side and wheeled to a recovery room where he or she is observed by nurses until fully conscious. When able to walk the patient returns to the ward and has a welcome cuppa and a snack (having fasted that morning as required before anaesthesia).

The most common after-effects include brief confusion, a dull headache and, after the first one or two treatments, pains in some muscle groups that are not accustomed to such activity.

The often-talked-about memory deficit, if it occurs at all, relates only to events occurring around the time of the treatment, not to established memories of the past. (Some patients hope that painful memories will be 'blotted out', and even mistakenly believe that this is the aim of the treatment.) Sophisticated psychological assessments have rarely found conclusive evidence of any permanent memory loss in recipients of ECT. To the contrary, tests show that memory often improves as a result of the remission of depression.

ECT is so safe that it can be given to a pregnant woman without risk to her or the foetus, and to people with high blood pressure, heart disease and peptic ulcers. Advanced age is no bar to treatment; seeing an aged person who has been languishing in a nursing home with a diagnosis of dementia regain their mental and physical faculties after a course of ECT is a rewarding experience.

There are only two conditions that rule out ECT treatment — brain tumour and a recent myocardial infarction (heart attack). ECT treatment of patients with other heart problems carries some risk, but to allow a severe agitated depression to continue in the presence of heart failure also carries a risk from the effect of over-exertion on the heart.

In keeping with today's high safety standards for people undergoing procedures under anaesthesia, comprehensive resuscitation equipment is present in the treatment room of a modern ECT suite. Since The Melbourne Clinic opened in 1978 over twelve thousand ECT treatments have been administered, and the resuscitation equipment has been needed only once — for a patient with pre-existing ischaemic heart disease (angina).

Treatments are usually carried out three times a week. The number of treatments required to ensure recovery varies. A good response is common after four to six treatments and another two are often given to minimise the chance of relapse. One young woman experienced complete remission after one treatment. Occasionally patients have prolonged courses when all other strategies have failed.

The biggest disadvantage of ECT, apart from the stigma, is that, unlike medication, it is given as a short course and then ceased. For this reason the rate of relapse within a short time is high. Some patients elect to have further treatments after recovery, at increasing intervals. This is because they have previously relapsed after ECT and medication has not been effective as a treatment for their depressive illness.

In less severe episodes of depression, where suicide is not a risk and the patient is not very severely impaired, there are alternative types of therapy. For all patients, supportive psychotherapy (with exploration of feelings, possible precipitating factors, and ongoing stresses in the patient's life) helps to restore the patient's self-esteem and lessen the chance of relapse.

Psychotherapies

The term *psychotherapy* refers to treatment by means of a dialogue and interaction between two people — a therapist and a patient (or client). There are many forms of psychotherapy, too many to cover in this book.

Not everyone requires specific types of psychotherapy; therapists regularly talking to patients are involved in psychotherapy, often called supportive psychotherapy. This title is not quite accurate, because therapists will often challenge the patient to make changes to current behaviour, rather than support them.

Successful therapy depends not on the specific type used but on finding a therapist who is effective, who inspires the patient's confidence and with whom the patient feels comfortable.

Two types of psychotherapy represent effective ways of helping to treat people with mood disorder (and other psychiatric problems). They are cognitive therapy, and dynamic psychotherapy, which is based on family therapy and psychodynamic models.

Cognitive Therapy

Dr Aaron Beck, an American psychiatrist, who found that traditional psychoanalytic-type treatment was not effective in his depressed patients, developed a treatment for depression known as cognitive psychotherapy, or cognitive behavioural psychotherapy. Some understanding of the processes of human development will give us an insight into what prompted his research.

The early 1970s saw the beginnings of approaches to mood disorder that dealt directly with the patient's thought processes (or cognitions).

This happened because therapists were working increasingly with people troubled by a variety of psychological or behavioural problems, not all of which were concrete, observable or measurable. These people were complaining of feeling anxious, miserable, unhappy, bored or frustrated, symptoms which occur commonly in people suffering from bipolar mood disorder. Yet, although these feelings were strong, they did not form a pattern indicating a serious psychological disorder. Often they merely prevented individuals from living in the way they would have preferred, because they had to avoid certain activities or because they were not achieving their goals or their potential. The problems were debilitating, but not to a degree requiring admission to a psychiatric hospital. In other cases the problem was simply that the person did not feel well, or happy, or confident, and they were seeking assistance to become happier or more fulfilled. Obviously modern psychology needed to move beyond areas of illness and pathological behaviour, and assist with problems of self-esteem, adjustment, feelings of malaise, anxiety, inappropriately high standards, lack of assertiveness, poor time management, and a myriad of more ordinary problems which most of us overcome.

With new findings on how we gather information and learn skills, whole new areas of psychological expertise developed, including stress management, social skills training, cognitive therapy, and endless variations of group experience as a path towards mental health. Traditional approaches to analytic therapy, such as psychoanalysis, had focused on a variety of mental events with the aim of providing insight, but the thinking or behavioural difficulties that pushed many clients into therapy often remained unchanged. Cognitive approaches, by contrast, introduced methods that worked on the thoughts themselves.

The combination of cognitive and behavioural methods was a powerful and flexible one with a number of advantages. Firstly, problems of happiness and adjustment could be treated — the 'suffering well' had somewhere to turn for help in adjusting to major or minor practical and personal issues. Secondly, many of these approaches could be formulated in such a way that non-trained people could apply them to their own difficulties without seeking professional help. Thus began the era of books and courses on effective psychological self-help. Cognitive therapy was available for people who wished to take control of their own lives. Where the problems were very distressing, or where they failed to respond to the available techniques, people could still fall back on the resources of an experienced therapist.

For someone suffering from acute and severe symptoms of a mood disorder, cognitive behavioural therapy (or CBT) is NOT a substitute for medical treatment. Applying psychologically-based techniques alone to acute symptoms is inappropriate and dangerous and can have very serious and potentially disastrous consequences.

Nevertheless, research and extensive clinical application have shown that CBT can make important contributions to the health and happiness of sufferers in three ways. Firstly, in the early stages, it can help them adjust to the knowledge that they have developed a severe and sometimes disruptive illness that might recur. Secondly, it can help them to manage difficulties created by the condition (irrational attitudes and negative self-beliefs often compound the problem). Finally, to the extent that upsetting events or stress can exacerbate the symptoms of mood disorder, the ongoing stress management provided by CBT can be of great value.

So what is CBT? Cognitive behavioural therapy approaches are based on the assumption that our emotional reactions are affected by the content of our thoughts. This directly reverses traditional medical attitudes that held that emotions directly create cognitions and therefore the alteration of mood is the most powerful way of influencing thinking.

The experimental evidence that thoughts influence emotion is compelling and largely stimulated by theories of Dr Aaron Beck and his colleagues. Experiments clearly demonstrated that mood can be immediately changed, becoming elevated or depressed respectively by the introduction of positive and negative ideas.

Such a causative process was recognised in the times of the Roman Empire when Epictetus, a Stoic philosopher, said that it was not the things that happen to us that upset us, but rather our view of these things.

This leads to the notion that we can change those thoughts that are distressing or dysfunctional for us. In other words, we have the potential to use cognitive therapy techniques to feel more comfortable, less distressed or less anxious.

However, feelings, even intensely uncomfortable ones, may be quite appropriate to the event that triggers them. For instance, if someone we love very much dies, it is appropriate for us to feel intense pain, anger and sadness. This grieving process helps us come to terms with losing an important person in our life. Where the relationship has been a very long and close one, the grieving person may experience some pain for the rest of their life, as often occurs when a spouse or child dies. The acute pain, desolation, anger and absorption with the loss will, however, diminish over time. Similarly, but taking a less traumatic example, if we have a day at work when everything goes wrong, most of us end up merely feeling frustrated. These feelings, while varying from uncomfortable to very painful, are appropriate to the situations both in the content and the intensity of the feeling. Appropriate feelings help us to adapt to our world and the events in which we are involved.

When an event is accompanied by feelings that are disproportionate to the event, we call the response *inappropriate.*

Consider the example of a young woman who has recently lost her mother. Imagine that she is very happily married with two well-adjusted young children whom she adores. We would expect her to miss her mother, with whom she had a strong bond of love and whose company she enjoyed immensely. It would not be unusual for her to withdraw socially and not to not feel like having fun. Periods of weeping, some anger about her mother's dying, recurring sadness, and a general loss of enjoyment would all be expected for a while, as part of the normal process of grieving. However, recovery from those feelings is likely to occur gradually and, in time — maybe six months, maybe twelve — she would probably be functioning as she did before her mother died. If, however, she believes that the future is hopeless and that life will never be good again without her mother, her mood is likely to continue to be depressed, to a greater degree, and for longer, than would be expected. Those particular beliefs are irrational and inappropriate to her situation, given her longstanding and happy family bonds. An unnecessary distress has been created by her beliefs.

It follows that irrational or inappropriate ideas are likely to be present where reactions to an event are excessive or unadaptive. If someone experiences incapacitating distress after an event which most people would find upsetting but not devastating, then it is likely that person thinks about the event differently from other people.

A corollary of this is that people can gain increased ability to cope in situations which incapacitate or distress them by examining the appropriateness or rationality of their ideas. By becoming aware of what they are saying to themselves, they may examine whether their views are appropriate, rational and adaptive and thus open the way to more adaptive thinking. Taking control of our unadaptive thinking in this way can enable us to get on with our life and reach our goals in a more effective way.

CBT provides a number of techniques for correcting thinking patterns perceived as unhelpful, even though they are also experienced as strongly believable.

The effectiveness of CBT for sufferers of mood disorder is best demonstrated by practical examples. We have put together a number of case studies of real situations that illustrate the solutions to some typical problems. CBT involves the use of various techniques, each chosen to suit the presenting problem in each case. Sometimes more than one CBT technique is used. The techniques described here are all suitable for readers to apply to any similar problems they might have. Where problems seem overwhelming or too difficult, professional help should be sought from a clinical psychologist.

Mrs C

Mrs C was very distressed by the fact that she suffered from bipolar disorder. This was not so much because of her experience and reactions to the condition as because of her fears about how people might react to her.

She had been briefly hospitalised after a manic episode and her mood difficulties had been treated successfully with medication. However, she felt ashamed that she had been in a psychiatric hospital and felt that her tennis club friends would never fully accept her again. She also believed that her very critical parents-in-law would have one more reason to condemn her marriage to their son and would make life even more difficult for her.

Technique 1: RET — Disputation

The approach used involves clarifying the belief system which an individual is applying to a particular situation or problem, and investigating its reality and logic. Based on the work of Albert Ellis, it is known as Rational Emotive Therapy (RET) — Disputation.

Application:

Mrs C was helped to 'spell out' why she felt so ashamed and afraid of rejection. Her assumption was that other people shared her belief that mental illness was stigmatising and a social disaster. She was asked for evidence that it was really awful and the worst catastrophe she could imagine. Thinking about it, she felt there were several other events she dreaded more. Having challenged her own 'awfulising' on this, she was able to accept a more rational view of her disorder as something she would rather not have, which was certainly very inconvenient and disruptive at times and a serious problem requiring help and good management. By viewing it in that light, rather than as a disaster, she felt less anxious about it and more able to take charge of its effect on her life.

She was then asked to consider the reality of her fears of rejection. Unable to come up with concrete examples of her friends' negative attitudes to mental illness, she realised she did not really know how they viewed such difficulties. She was encouraged to remember how she had viewed such psychological problems before she had needed psychiatric help, and how she had changed her views with recently acquired knowledge. It was quite possible that her tennis friends, even if they were negative, might respond to some clear facts about the condition when she told them what had been happening to her. She was also reminded that the club had sent flowers and several well-wishing cards. She was able to compare it to the continuing, unambiguously negative behaviour of her in-laws and realised that she had been 'mind-reading', rather than basing her conclusions on clear evidence from her friends.

She was also asked to think about why the possibility or actuality of social rejection hurt her. She responded that, if someone rejected her, that meant she was not likeable, was not a good person. When confronted with the evidence of others who did like her and thought she was a good person, she laughingly had to agree such an absolute generalisation drawn from rejection by one or two people was not logical. She came to agree that any person was free to reject her or approve of her, but that such opinion was not the sole determinant of her likeability or worth. Although it was unfortunate that her in-laws disapproved, she agreed that she was not defined by their opinions of her, and consequently felt less distressed by that issue.

Sometimes, this kind of disputing of irrational beliefs needs to be done many times, because the ideas may keep recurring, particularly if they are long-standing. To be effective, a repetitive, propaganda-type approach might work best, and perhaps in a structured format. We have included here an RET worksheet filled out by Mrs C. She did this exercise every day, taking for her subject the day's most uncomfortable situation or thought. The following example shows her dealing with her response to an upsetting incident with her in-laws.

Technique 2: Behavioural Assignment

It can be very powerful, when attempting to change irrational beliefs, to go further than just challenging beliefs in an intellectual way. A technique used to change attitudes, known as Behavioural Assignment, might include doing a task that will clarify the reality of our assumptions or expose us to an alternative and more rational viewpoint. Having a model of how someone else copes can show us, very concretely, an alternative way of thinking and acting from which we can learn new responses.

Application:

Mrs C was encouraged to contact a woman she had met in hospital, whom she admired, and to ask her how she felt about the stigma of having psychiatric difficulties. When they talked this woman related her own experiences, which included being rejected briefly by her teenage son while she was in hospital. She recognised her son's fear of being stigmatised by his mother's hospitalisation, and helped him with it. In doing so, she reaffirmed her own view that her illness was not of her choosing. She had come to accept it, without apology or anger, and now put her emotional energy into living a life that was as fulfilling as possible, rather than focusing that energy negatively on her illness.

Mrs C then decided to carry out a second behavioural assignment, and went back to her tennis club, rather than continue to avoid it. She was able to report that everybody had been very warm and those she knew better had been actively interested in details of her recovery. Two women there told her that they, too, had received psychiatric treatment after the birth of their babies.

Mr D

Mr D suffered from recurrent major depression. He stated that he felt anxious and confused. He asked for help in clarifying his problems, which he had spent hours worrying about without ever resolving anything.

Technique: Problem Listing

There is a simple strategy which is useful when we become so immersed in our difficulties that we lose a sense of perspective, and every new issue becomes an additional source of anxiety. We list all the possible problems, then group related problems together. This allows questions to be asked which give perspective, such as:

- What are the problems most needing a solution right now?
- Which problems are going to be the most disruptive in one month, or six months, or five years?
- Which problem, if I solved it right now, would make the most positive difference?
- Which problems are within my power to solve?
- Which problems require problem solving or practical action, and which require me to change my thinking?

Application:
Time was allocated to help Mr D describe all his worries, which were then presented back to him in a list. The next step was to see which problems appeared closely related, and then decide which presented the most difficulty immediately, and in the long term. To his surprise it seemed that he had no immediate difficulties, apart from some issues which he judged as minor. His major worries were focused on the future, centred around his perceived inability to make plans. He felt that anything he undertook might be disrupted by a breakdown. This affected planning for holidays, trips overseas with his wife, his wish to apply for promotion and his knowledge that it would be good for his health if he joined a gymnasium. By this time, he felt much less anxious because he had been able to define his problems more clearly, which also showed him that many parts of his life caused him no problems.

An analysis of Mr D's problem list showed up the following specific aspects:

- He overreacted to any small signs of depression or change in his coping ability, assuming that another descent into major depression had begun.
- He felt anxious about bothering his doctor over his concerns and previously had sought help only when his mood was very depressed.
- He felt he could not stand another breakdown and hated the idea of returning to the hospital where he had been briefly admitted when his condition first became acutely obvious.

These issues were discussed at length with Mr D using the RET technique. After discussion, he was able to appreciate that his anxieties were fuelled by ideas that he could identify as irrational. However, he said that he could see things that way only with his therapist present. Otherwise he felt completely unable to challenge any thoughts when he was depressed or anxious, even if he attempted to use the RET exercise format described earlier. A technique to provide him with easier access to rational thinking was required.

Technique: Cognitive Propaganda Cards
The person's typical irrational beliefs or thought processes are identified and understood as such, and counteracting rational

statements are recorded on what we call Cognitive Propaganda Cards. These may be written singly or as a list on a conveniently sized card or sheet of paper, and read at pre-determined frequency for example, three times daily or when events occur that create emotional distress or worry.

Application:
Mr D was asked to read the statements below twice daily (on the train to and from work, and before breakfast and dinner at the weekends). He was also to read the cards when he felt any depressive symptoms. Each statement was written on one side of small index cards which fitted into his suit pocket.

CARD 1
Most people experience minor changes of mood each day. The majority of my mood changes over the last year have been minor, occurring after something happened to which I reacted fairly normally and lasting for a short time.

CARD 2
If I do become clinically depressed, I will deal with that when it happens. After all, I have already worked out good plans with my wife and my doctor in case that does happen. So it is fruitless and unnecessary to worry.

CARD 3
Questions I should ask myself if I think I am becoming depressed:

1 Am I strongly depressed?
2 Is there no concrete reason for how I am feeling?
3 Has this feeling lasted longer than it would for someone else in similar circumstances?

Three 'yes' answers mean I should talk to my wife about what I am feeling and together we can decide whether I ought to see the doctor. Less than three means I am worrying unnecessarily.

CARD 4
Major depression has in fact occurred only twice in my life and my tendency toward this is being kept under control by medication. So, although it is very disruptive and distressing when it does occur, I need to remember that it is not frequent.

CARD 5
Having a major depressive episode is upsetting, very disruptive

and highly unpleasant. However I CAN stand it, as I have before.

CARD 6
My doctor is there to help me. Therefore it is OK to ask him or advice when I am worried. I have a lot to gain from doing that, because if I am becoming depressed, we can do something about it in the early stages. It is not the worst thing in the world to see him, even if we discover that I was worrying unnecessarily. And if he thinks I am going too often, he can be assertive and tell me.

However, Mr D was unsure how supportive his doctor really was. Anticipating that he would still find it difficult to approach him when he was feeling down he decided to check it out.

Technique: Practical Problem Solving
Changing one's thinking can be important but sometimes a situation requires practical problem solving in order to make the situation better.

Application:
Mr D decided to talk to his doctor and tell him that he would feel more supported if he knew that the doctor would not object if sometimes he came in just to check his symptoms. He explained that he would rather sometimes come unnecessarily than feel anxious at home. If his doctor had been unsympathetic about this, he planned to change doctors, finding one who met his emotional need for support, in addition to his medical needs. Fortunately his doctor responded well.

Part of Mr D's dread of relapsing was his dislike of the hospital to which he had been admitted. This was the only local State hospital. He decided that, should he require hospitalisation for his condition in the future, he would prefer admission to another local hospital, which was private. Mr D joined a private health insurance scheme, taking top cover. The pre-existing illness clause meant that he was not covered for hospitalisation in the event of depression for twelve months. However, he knew that the prospect of hospitalisation would be less distressing for him after that waiting period had elapsed.

Mr N
For fifteen years, Mr N had been treated for episodes of depression. The last episode had followed a major change in his life,

when he retired from his job which had absorbed all his energy. Usually he recovered from a relapse fairly quickly. This time was different. He was no longer clearly depressed or suicidal but just did not have any energy or ability to organise himself. He stayed at home watching television and his wife complained that he was grumpy and bored. His friends were all still at work, most of them some years away from retirement.

He described himself as being in a rut, and having little staying power in trying new activities. He was easily frustrated and tired quickly, becoming very cross at himself. Recognising that he needed a structure to help him get going again, he asked for some ideas on how to go about this.

Technique: Graduated Activity Scheduling

It is important to understand why activities are not being completed. Where the reasons include mild depression, habit, poor discipline or inappropriately high goals, graduated activity scheduling offers an appropriate solution. It involves creating a list of activities that the person would like to do and determining for each activity the current difficulty or the likelihood of completion for that person. It may need to be combined with other techniques or medical treatment if other factors such as high anxiety, assertion problems or illness are the reason for inactivity.

Goals are set initially at a level very close to the current level of achievement, in both frequency and difficulty, and in line with the person's own assessment of what is most achievable. Goals and achievements are recorded so that gains are not taken for granted and serve as a source of reinforcement, particularly when progress is slow.

Goals need to be reviewed regularly. Where success in a particular activity is being achieved at goal level, then the level may be increased if desired, or maintained at that level, with a decrease in the conscious effort required to do so. Goals may be dropped when they become irrelevant, whether or not they are being met.

Application:

Mr N drew up a list of things he wanted to be able to do as part of a normal week. Activities chosen included exercise, social activities, hobbies and household tasks. He then chose four activities from that list and concentrated on establishing those activities as regular parts of his week. Recognising that he had been doing very little in any of those areas, he set modest goals. This also gave him a chance to build up his confidence and perseverance. He achieved all of his goals in the first week. He walked around the block twice, telephoned a friend, had a haircut and dropped in once at the local pub.

The following week, he maintained his walking at the same level because he had found even that difficult, but he increased his social contact goals. He continued to be flexible in increasing the level expected each week, depending on his success and on his enjoyment of the activity. New activities were added in as he felt able to handle them.

Before using these techniques, Mr N had often become frustrated and depressed when he attempted a task. If success did not come immediately, he usually gave up. The therapy encouraged him to view 'failure' not as devastating evidence of the impossibility of achieving the task but as part of a process of trial and error which contributed to learning. 'Failures' became statements about whether the size of the step taken is appropriate, whether the goal was appropriate, and how to approach the task more successfully. Mr N became more tolerant of setbacks which in turn helped him get over a period of illness which kept him in bed for several weeks.

With all his friends still working, Mr N then decided that he needed to widen his social network. Graduated activity scheduling gave him some ideas about how to structure this change.

Technique: Setting up Networks

We depend on those around us for much of our emotional, social, informational and practical support. Most of us are surrounded by family, friends and relatives who love and nurture us, share time and talk things over with us, help us when we have problems, and tell us how to get things done. This is our social network.

Relationships within our networks vary in closeness, quality, activities shared, and so on. Such variety is important as we develop our network to support our own diverse needs. Having a network which suits us contributes to our feeling of fulfilment and helps us manage better in times of stress. If our lives, or the lives of others who are very significant to us, undergo major changes, we might need to develop new networks or refine the ones we have in order to accommodate the change. Events that commonly create this need to change our social networks include retirement, a sudden major disability, having a baby, moving to another city, and beginning study in a new setting.

For most of us, however, building a social network in the first place involved very little conscious effort. This can create a problem when major rebuilding of a network is required. The three main principles for developing better social networks described by psychologists Fensterheim and Baer are therefore very useful. They are:

- Start where you are — look at the possibilities already existing in your life. Even the most isolated person has some sort of contact with other human beings. Build on the contacts you have.
- Maintain a step-by-step progression towards your goals.
- Constantly experiment with your network and continue making improvements.

Application:
Incorporating these activities into his weekly goal program, Mr N looked at his current social possibilities in terms of what they might offer, rather than what they did not provide. He then chose to follow up a number of distant acquaintances, arranging to meet them, or going out of his way to chat when he saw them in his local pub. He had never been much of a drinker, but saw the social possibilities of such a venue. Over several months, he became very friendly with three people there and began joining them on regular fishing trips. At the same time, he was pursuing an avenue entirely new to him — he joined a political club — and this gave a whole new range of acquaintances. Two very close friendships developed there and he and his wife spent many happy social occasions with these new friends and their wives. He continued to see his old friends during the weekends and felt that he had achieved a balance that met his retirement needs.

Mrs W
Mrs W was managing her mood disorder well, and was generally happy and confident. However, she reported being stressed and overloaded from time to time, often suffering tension headache.

When she described her daily life, it became obvious that she was doing too much. Although she was efficient, she simply did not have enough time for everything she wanted to achieve. She was attempting to be on hand for her three children as much as she had been before she took up a full-time job. In addition, she expected to keep her house immaculate, be involved in community groups, help her aged mother and still be fresh, attractive and ready for socialising with her husband in the evening.

Technique 1: Time Management

Managing our time well gives us control over our lives. No one else is in such a good position to do this and no one has so much to gain.

The first step in time management is to identify long-term goals for ourselves, not forgetting to list the less material goals such as having a quality family life and a healthy lifestyle.

Then we need to list lots of possible activities that we might do in the immediate term that will assist our progress towards these goals. In other words, what can we do now, this week? We can then put a priority on each activity on the list that will contribute to achieving our goals. Low-priority items (those that contribute little to our long-term goals) can be eliminated.

The next step is to schedule time for the high-priority items in the coming week. Time needs to be blocked out for each activity. For time management to work, the schedule must be adhered to.

Another useful technique is to pick a priority for any given time, and ask yourself what is the most productive use of this time right now? Consult your list of long-term goals and current chosen activities for guidance.

Managing time well frees us up to make spontaneous choices and to respond to opportunities that might suddenly arise, while providing assurance that the important activities for the week are attended to.

Application:

Mrs W drew up a list of everything she wanted to do in the following week and rated these activities in order of priority for achieving her long-term goals. She included goals such as sleeping, resting and relaxation, which were important for her stress management, which in turn was essential for progress towards her long-term goals. Top-priority activities were scheduled and low priority activities scratched, though Mrs W reported having trouble doing that. Having checked the end result of her plan again, she proceeded to try it out. Problems did occur with her seemingly automatic tendency to respond to all requests and try to do everything that came up.

However, she persevered, gradually finding herself making decisions thoughtfully, and undoing a number of arrangements she had entered into which, on reflection, she decided were in conflict with her own priorities. Thus, she became better at protecting her time for her priorities rather than bowing to other people's. She also felt much more satisfied with her level of achievement.

In concentrating less on 'busyness' and more on the quality of results, she came to put a higher value on some of the aesthetic and pleasurable parts of her life. Her sex life improved and she began listening to music more often.

Technique 2: Relaxation

People who are anxious, depressed or under stress often feel tense physically or complain of being unable to switch off. Various effective methods of relaxation have been developed to assist this problem. Time-honoured methods of unwinding, such as having a rest, stopping for a chat, going for a walk or a run, and watching a sunset should not be forgotten and should be included in the lives of all of us.

There are many ways of reducing tension. The most common include:

- Muscle relaxation. This can be progressive, focussing on all the muscle groups in the body one at a time or more globally, including whole body stretches or flopping. This process can include tensing and then relaxing the muscles, or simply focussing on the muscles and letting them relax. Such a technique can be very effectively combined with day-to-day activities (such as washing dishes), as these often prompt unnecessary muscle tension in themselves.
- Breathing exercises. These include consciously breathing at a slightly slower rate, breathing to empty the lungs more, use of the more sophisticated yoga breathing techniques and breathing in conjunction with imagery. Examples of this include imagining the tension as a dark colour and visualising the colour being breathed out into the air,

leaving a lighter colour in the body.

- Visual imagery. Thinking of pleasant peaceful images — perhaps a beach, a safe comfortable place, a flickering candle or a beautiful cloud — help produce a more tranquil frame of mind and can provide an antidote and block to a constant stream of worrying images or stressful thoughts.

Initially relaxation needs to be practised in a stress-free, peaceful environment. Like any skill, mastery comes with regular practice. Twice-daily sessions of at least twenty minutes are advised. After a few weeks of practice, relaxation may be carried out in brief episodes and in busier and more stressful situations. By then, it is a very useful anti-stress tool which can be used to counteract and diminish stress exactly when it is occurring.

Application:
Because Mrs W was experiencing tension headaches, she chose to use a progressive muscle relaxation approach. Twice daily, once during a twenty-minute morning bath, and once lying down on her bed for half an hour after returning from work, she concentrated in turn on each part of her body, letting tension go from each. She then did a tension/relaxation exercise on parts of her body that were still tense. She paid particular attention to her neck, jaw and face. Then she imagined scenes from her last holiday on a beautiful tropical beach.

Within a week she reported that her headaches had gone and that she felt more energetic. She also enjoyed the relaxation practice immensely, taught it to her family and decided to have a professional massage once a week as well.

Dynamic Psychotherapy

At birth we painfully and suddenly emerge into a world very different from the protection of the womb. We grow rapidly for the first fifteen or so years and also face many years of schooling before being accepted as an adult.

We need to make friends, find suitable employment and move away from home and family. In time we might find a lover and go on to have a family of our own. At some stage we have to face the illness and death of those close to us, and in turn others will have to cope with our death.

All this in the space of six to eight decades.

Being human can be difficult. Crises occur, relationships

fracture, major disappointments arise. Through this, our internal world — the world of feelings, thoughts and imagination that we recognise as our inner self — can be plunged into turmoil. Slowly we reassert ourselves and, slowly, equilibrium returns. If we are fortunate there is an understanding friend to encourage and assist us, but there are times when our inner world can be rocked to its very foundations — when we are overwhelmed with sadness or despair, grasping at fragments of an inner chaos, tumbling alone in a void. In time we may even turn against our inner world, precipitating an inner split, an abyss separating self from self.

In desperation we seek a guide; but this time more than friendship is required. This time the guide will be required to join with us to form a healing relationship, a relationship which will enable us either to rediscover our inner integrity or to build it anew.

The guide might be a friend or a lover, as before; but more usually this guide is someone who has undertaken an apprenticeship in being a guide to others. Such a person may be a psychotherapist, and the healing relationship offered is then called psychotherapy.

Dynamic psychotherapy aims to help develop self-awarenes and emotional resilience. By using the patient–psychotherist relationship as a model for other relationships, it encourages patients to cope with painful feelings that they might otherwise block from their awareness and to make connections which enable unhelpful repetitive patterns of behaviour to dissolve.

Individuals with a mood disorder are likely to have feelings of rejection, sadness and grief, and to have particular difficulty coping with times of separation and loss.

Dynamic psychotherapy is indicated when there are particular or repeated difficulties negotiating situations in which these feelings emerge.

As with cognitive therapy, the complexity and effectiveness of dynamic psychotherapy are best demonstrated by examples drawn from real situations. The cases are amalgams and significant personal details have been changed to ensure confidentiality.

Rebecca

Rebecca was twenty-two and studying Arts at university. When referred by her local doctor for psychotherapy, she had been depressed for two months.

Rebecca confided that she had recently discontinued an

unsatisfactory relationship which had dragged on for almost eighteen months. On reflection, she felt that she had probably endured the relationship because it had offered her an opportunity to leave home, which she had felt pressured by her family to do. Although convinced that ending the relationship was the right course to take, she now felt lost and alone.

Rebecca spoke of a long-standing dispute with her younger sister, Tina, and with her parents. For as long as she could remember she had felt that her parents had rejected her in favour of Tina and that she had been treated unfairly. Rebecca resented the fact that her parents seemed always ready to see Tina's point of view but never hers. She insisted that she was continually and unfairly blamed when household chores were left undone. Her deepest resentment, however, was that her parents seemed to show little interest in her.

Unhappy at home and isolated socially, Rebecca became increasingly depressed despite the support of her therapist. Her capacity to concentrate and to study effectively was becoming impaired and she became troubled by suicidal thoughts. A course of tricyclic antidepressants was commenced and over the next few weeks her mood and outlook improved.

Rebecca decided to take a holiday interstate, where she met a young man, Michael, who shared her musical interests. They soon developed a close relationship. Although very fond of Michael, Rebecca was distressed to find jealous feelings emerging. It was obvious to Rebecca that Michael was reciprocating her attention and affection, yet she held a deep, underlying fear that his primary attention was elsewhere and that she would soon be rejected. Despite outward evidence that the relationhip was progressing well, Rebecca could not put fears of impending rejection from her mind and again began to feel depressed. Disputes with her family at home worsened, and Rebecca and her therapist decided to hold a meeting with them.

Rebecca's parents were eager to attend and shared *their* distress at being unable to resolve disputes between Tina and Rebecca. They acknowledged feeling overprotective of Tina but felt that this protection was necessary because of what they regarded as Rebecca's domineering behaviour at home. Tina, in turn, harboured deep resentments in relation to Rebecca, whom she saw as thoughtlessly pursuing her own interests regardless of Tina's welfare.

In discussion it transpired that Rebecca had been a much-loved first child, doted on by her mother until three years old, when Tina was born. Tina had respiratory problems at birth and for two years her parents were uncertain that she would survive. Tina required constant attention day and night and Rebecca's mother recalled profound concern that Rebecca was being short changed and missing appropriate parental attention.

Animated family discussion followed as a possible explanation for the long-standing rivalry and jealousy between Rebecca and her sister emerged. Her parents could also see that over-protectiveness of Tina had persisted and was no longer appropriate.

Although dispute within the family continued, Rebecca felt that she now understood its deeper roots and somehow was better able to manage. She also felt that her parents were now more ready to listen to her point of view and that both she and Tina were better placed to negotiate rather than retreat defensively.

Following the family session, Rebecca's mood lifted considerably and she was clearly less troubled by feelings of rejection and abandonment. Significantly, she felt more at ease in her relationship with Michael and was able to reassure herself (or be reassured by Michael) when fear of rejection arose.

Helen

When Helen first came to see her family therapist she was fifty-five years of age and had been suffering from severe depression for most of the preceding six years. She had been admitted to hospital on several occasions following suicide attempts and had gained only limited relief from a variety of antidepressant medications and a course of electroconvulsive therapy.

Helen was a practising Catholic. She relished the task of parenting her three children, and they had been brought up strictly within the faith and without great difficulty until her eldest daughter, Sarah, who was nineteen, became seriously involved with a boy whom Helen described as an atheist.

Helen and her husband intervened, insisting that Sarah break off the relationship. To Helen's horror Sarah left home and set up flat with her boyfriend. A rift developed between Sarah and her parents and over the next three years her two remaining daughters also left home, essentially cutting off ties with their parents.

At the time of referral, Helen appeared overwhelmed with despair. She was convinced that her children had rejected her and that she had failed as a parent. There was also another source of distress and bitterness. She felt she had failed her church and had been let down by her faith.

After Helen and her family therapist had talked, it was decided that a family meeting would be set up. In fact, five family meetings approximately six weeks apart were to occur over a period of eight months.

When the family met it was actually the first time they had all been together for six years. This first session was particularly moving as Helen tearfully explained to Sarah in front of the family why she and her husband had intervened in her relationship six years previously.

Sarah, in turn, was able to tell of her anguish when she was confronted with having to choose between her boyfriend and her family. She had become married to the same young man soon after the separation and now they had two young children.

In the early family sessions it became possible for Helen, Sarah and her other two daughters to accept each other again. It also became apparent that far from being failures as parents, Helen and her husband had actually been very successful in that each of the children had left home, married happily and were actively engaged in living fulfilling lives.

Soon a different theme emerged in the sessions: Helen's lifelong struggle for independence. This struggle had persisted since her early days of restrictive convent education and had continued up until the present time.

In fact, it emerged that Helen and her daughters were not so very different from each other in their desire for independence. It also became clear to Helen that her own struggle with the restrictions imposed by her education was a struggle shared by many others. Slowly a dawning awareness emerged for Helen that she really was not alone.

Within the family, Helen's struggle came to be seen as a struggle of heroic dimensions, from which the family had painfully emerged. Far from being a failure, Helen had been at the forefront of this struggle. To some extent Helen's daughters were further along the way than herself and could perhaps now give her a lead.

A significant aspect of the family sessions was the assistance it gave Helen to 'put herself together again'. Helen had been experiencing a profound sense of inner fragmentation following both the separation from her daughters and the struggle she was having with her faith.

In the final two sessions Helen was able to speak of a new sense of self emerging. At first there were only glimpses of this but in the presence of her family it was as if she were able to retrieve a number of lost parts of herself and put these missing bits of the jigsaw back together again. For the first time in some years she began to see herself as a whole person. Helen spoke with emotion of this experience, which had been both painful and frightening for her. Perhaps, in biblical terms, she was experiencing her resurrection.

Helen's depression and despair lifted considerably after the family sessions. Subsequently she engaged in a re-negotiation of her relationship with her faith with the help of a supportive priest.

Tom

Tom is thirty-two years old, with a history of multiple admissions to public psychiatric hospitals over a period of several years, first beginning at age twenty-six. On most of these occasions Tom was extremely high.

For some years he was treated with major tranquillisers and lithium before being referred to his current psychiatrist for psychotherapy.

Tom struggled to find some meaning in these experiences.

Whilst his psychiatrist was on holidays Tom was admitted to hospital in a highly suspicious state. He thought that a jar of relish that had been placed on the coffee table before him contained a 'bug' (that is, a microphone).

Later his therapist offered him the following interpretation:

When the psychiatrist was on holidays Tom felt that he had been abandoned and that nobody cared for him. The 'little boy' inside him found this state of abandonment so difficult to cope with that he conjured up a fantasy for himself which ensured that Tom was the centre of attention. The fantasy was that he was of acute interest to everybody around him. Even jars of relish had microphones in them to ensure that Tom's every word was noticed.

Tom needed to recognise that such fantasies were themselves expressions of emotions. If he could get in touch with these emotions he would not need to take the fantasy literally.

For example, if he had noted that he was insecure in his psychiatrist's absence and coped with this he could have reassured himself that his therapist would return before long. Instead of this he bought his own fantasy wholesale, which prevented him, as an adult, from dealing with the issues concerned.

Together he and his therapist drew parallels between this process and what had occurred when he was with friends in Queensland at the time of his first breakdown. Tom had never been away from his family before and whilst travelling with two companions he had become intensely frightened in Brisbane, necessitating his return home and subsequent admission to a psychiatric hospital. At that time, as on this admission, he had also developed intense fears that he had become the focus of everybody's attention.

Tom was very keen to ensure that he did not lapse into fantasy again, and he and his therapist agreed to work together to give him some guidelines that would help achieve this.

Using a whiteboard and some felt pens Tom and his therapist began to list the differences between fantasy and reality. The result is outlined in the table on the following page.

As Tom talked with his therapist he became increasingly aware of the richness of his own imagination and of how creative he could be. He remarked on how successful he had been in a singing role in an amateur stage production. Nevertheless his capacity to imagine frightened him and he tried to enlist his psychiatrist's support to suppress it.

Instead his therapist encouraged him to try harder to distinguish between fantasy and real experience. In order for this to occur he would also need to learn how to focus (and refocus) his attention on real-life experience and actively guard against being distracted by fantasies, no matter how impelling. If he could become more skilful at seeing the difference then perhaps his imagination could become an enricher of his real experience in life rather than a distraction repeatedly demanding enactment.

As mentioned earlier, Tom had been taking lithium and major tranquillisers for some time. Psychotherapy can and often does proceed hand in hand with the use of medication. In fact, the medication available today often allows psychotherapy (including family therapy) to proceed in situations where this would have not been possible in the past.

There are also situations in which psychotherapy has to be

FANTASY Bizarre Nonsense No limits to the imagination (Anything I imagine or think about is possible)	**REALITY** Not bizarre Commonsense Reality has limits (e.g. society's laws, religious (moral) laws, laws of physics/nature, laws of probability)
HIGH ('Clayton's' happiness) No one else is laughing Feedback from others might not be positive and might be negative Brittle — turns quickly to anger/sadness/anxiety Inhuman Belittling Doesn't settle but escalates	**REAL HAPPINESS** Others are laughing Feedback from other people encouraging and positive Hearty deep-felt laugh — not euphoric — not brittle Humanity maintained Settles easily

put on hold (apart from encouragement and support) until medication has had time to take effect. This happens when the individual is too unsettled and unwell to take in and benefit from the psychotherapeutic experience.

Another patient, Gina, became bogged down in her therapy and no progress was being made. Such 'sticking points' are not unusual in psychotherapy, but this particular case seemed totally hopeless. Gina was prescribed antidepressants and, within three weeks, her despair had lifted. She was clearly less depressed, once again there was some hope, and the work with her therapist began to take on a new dimension.

If psychotherapy is helpful, it might be possible to reduce medication and in time, hopefully, do without it. However, whilst this is a reasonable goal, it is not always achievable.

The psychotherapist might cautiously recommend adjustments to medication, according to progress in therapy. Sometimes, however, the medication is being prescribed by another psychiatrist or doctor. In such cases psychotherapy can proceed quite satisfactorily, providing reasonable agreement is reached between the parties concerned.

Psychotherapy can be a brief or a lengthy experience. Rebecca's therapist will probably never hear from her again; whereas Helen and her husband might renew contact from time to time. Tom is likely to continue to be in therapy for some years to come.

The Aftermath of Treatment

The aftershocks following the 'earthquake' of mania continue for some time after the initial disturbance has settled; and patients who have been in the deep, dark pit of depression suffer long after they have come back to the light of a balanced life. Of course, every individual varies in the speed and extent of their response to treatment.

For those who have suffered their first attack, there is the prospect of coming to terms with having a biological illness, and the possible need for long-term, even life-long, medication. If the attack has been a recurrence — for example, following a decision to cease lithium maintenance therapy — the experience may be salutary, particularly for those who have had a manic episode in which they suffered financial, social or family disaster for the second time. If the episode has occurred in spite of ongoing treatment, it is a time for reassessment by the patient and psychiatrist, in whom the patient's trust might be understandably shaken. For all patients there is the likelihood of feelings of inadequacy, horror, self-reproach or fear. Guilt feelings are common. The post-treatment period is a very fragile time during which they might have difficulty forgiving themselves.

It takes a long time to lose the memories of such a disaster and become integrated again in the community. Some people have the ability to block out most of the experiences of illness, though this is not necessarily healthy, particularly if it leads to making the same mistake again.

Yet for many people the memories are not all bad. Certainly people who have experienced mania remember with some pleasure the feelings of omnipotence and infallibility; and, perhaps surprisingly, some people who have suffered the depths of depression also recall positive aspects of the experience which enabled them to get in touch with areas of themselves that had been obscured by the defence mechanisms of the mind. Some patients describe the experience of psychosis as having elements related to a previously undeveloped spirituality. With sensitive psychiatric help, all of these positive aspects of the illness can be put to good use in the healing process.

Many psychiatrists now perceive a person wholistically; that is, they view the person as having emotional, physical, mental and spiritual needs to attend to. Until these are fully rehabilitated and harmonised within the person who has suffered mood disorder, some imbalances or insecurities might remain. A psychiatrist, psychologist, social worker or nurse can provide counselling that enables these needs to be answered and a feeling of completeness to be achieved.

Careers or occupations need to be restored, competencies in relating to people re-established, a faith in existence and the meaning of life encouraged, confidence in personal abilities fostered, and a positive attitude towards engaging in creative and recreational pursuits revived. This total approach is termed wholistic healing.

Since we live in a competitive society, re-adjustment can be quite a battle for some. Whatever the level of adjustment, the recovered patient is still vulnerable and needs considerable understanding and support.

However, as the testimonies in this book so vividly show, the prospects for full recovery are, in most cases, very good.

Donna

'There is a block about mental illness in society but there isn't a block in my head as much as there was.'

I think my grandfather had a significant influence on my life. He was a very gentle man and appeared to understand me a lot. I felt at the time that my father had sort of rejected me. He was very tough on me, and so I suppose I turned to my grandfather for what I probably should have got from my father.

I understand it more now. My father was an alcoholic but he didn't recognise it. I don't think any of us did until quite a way down the track. I was well and truly married by then, and I would say that had a bearing on my feelings towards him and alcohol. I think my grandfather saw what was happening, and he and I were drawn together. He had a lot of time for me. Whereas my father used to tell me to concentrate harder and do better at school, my grandfather spent time with me, teaching me the things that I had difficulty with, and I seemed to do very well under his patience and teaching.

I would say that both my grandparents on my mother's side, and my mother, had a great influence on me, too. Mother is an incredible woman. She has a backbone like a steel spring. No matter what happens she can bounce back, or appears to. I think she had a very happy young life before she got married, but when she got married — as Dad started to drink — I think it became very difficult for her, both financially and emotionally. He was a beautiful man out of drink, but in drink he was unbelievable. I had to physically tear him off my mother because he would be brutal. In fact, one time, at about fifteen or sixteen, I tried to kill him, and I have always felt that one of my roles in life was to protect my mother. I always feel like that, still. But I forgive my father now, because he rehabilitated himself, and he was brilliant in his field. He was a Doctor of Dentistry. He felt guilty as well when I appeared to become ill. Unkindly poor thing, he used to joke about me being 'schizo', but he didn't want to know about it.

My sister had a mental breakdown — I suppose at about fifteen or sixteen. It was depression. But I wouldn't say that she was manic-depressive at all. She overcame whatever it was. I think it was perhaps Dad's condition. She was a loner at school, and she was a big girl and had trouble finding out who she was. We didn't have any teenage life, really. We were trying to hide the fact that our father drank. Mum used to say he had a practice to attend. It didn't matter whether the sky fell in during the weekend, on Monday morning you went out that front door as if nothing had happened, and you didn't tell anybody. So we had a lot of stuff that we had to keep inside ourselves.

I now realise that is why I had difficulty at school myself. I had difficulty concentrating, because I never knew, when I turned the corner, what I was coming home to. That went on for years, so it must have affected us both, even though there are six years between us. Quite honestly I couldn't, in a way, wait to leave home. I didn't think of it in terms of leaving home, I thought of it in terms of getting married and leaving home. I felt I needed to be protected.

My father-in-law and my husband didn't believe that

women should go out to work. So I got my rewards from motherhood, and I have always felt it a wonderful reward to work in a domestic capacity. It is up to you whether you make it that. You cannot do two jobs properly. I don't think there are enough people who think about it hard enough today.

I didn't go out to work until my youngest was eighteen. I had sworn to myself that, one day, when Antonia was eighteen, I would do something for myself, and that is exactly what I did, twenty-eight years down the track. But I wouldn't have done it if my therapist hadn't one day got a little agitated with me, and said, 'You should be selling something,' and I thought, 'What the hell is he on about?' I came home and I thought, 'Well, I am going to get myself togged up, because I would love to be a sales assistant.' That's really what I had wanted to do all those years ago. I went out and I got the second job that I went for.

I became a sales assistant, in women's fashion, and I stayed there only six months because I found it too far to drive from where I live. I got a bit anxious, actually, and one of the signs when I get anxious is that I have difficulty driving — my legs seem to go. I found myself driving with trucks around me and I couldn't handle that at all. I thought, 'This is a wasted exercise. I'm putting myself through hell and it's not really worth it.' So I left and did some figure work for my husband at home, and for the past twelve months I've been working in a dress shop. I love it, but I only work part time because I also love my two days at home. I'm very much, if you like, a Jewish mama, although I'm not Jewish. I think a family is very important.

My husband started to notice instability in me. I didn't. He felt that it was possibly due to the life I'd had at home. He felt that there was something wrong, without knowing exactly what. Obviously I was having mood swings then. I'd be unreasonable, wanting to spend twenty-four hours a day with him, and I suppose I was frustrated because I wasn't really allowed to go out to work. I really wanted a baby, but I couldn't have one until three years down the track. Once I'd had a baby, then the whole world changed for me again, and that was great, but I wasn't content with one — I wanted another one. We couldn't have any more ourselves, so we adopted one and then another. As long as I had babies to look after I was happy and I suppose I felt justified in being at home. I loved it. I enjoyed every minute of those babies, even when they started growing up.

I was very, very plump, and I used to really want to be skinny, like a model. So I went to a GP and I got some slimming tablets. I took them for a long time, and I had endless energy. I used to paint at night till one or two in the morning, and I could live on very little sleep. Obviously they gave me a high. I took those on and off for years, but not increasing the dose. That was the beginning of the end if you like. I'd been taking them and they used to make me feel suicidal. I used to dream of drowning in water or running away, because I obviously wasn't handling the situation I was in at all. I thought I was, but I wasn't.

I needed counselling then. I had a little bit of it, but one fellow said to me, 'Why the hell don't you do something?' and I thought 'I don't know what he's talking about.' Nobody would ever sit down and talk to me in depth about anything. Another counsellor I went to said, 'I know what you want, and I'm not giving it to you.' And he would sit there through all these sessions not talking, so I wouldn't talk either. I thought that was a waste of money. Then Stephen brought a car that he wanted to do up, and I was furious and took an overdose of Valium. I was sent to the Alfred Hospital. After that I had counselling on and off.

After this episode I felt tired all the time. All the slimming tablets had been taken away from me, and all I wanted really was slimming tablets to get me back up on a really big high like I'd been having. I wasn't coping psychologically at all. Then I went somewhere else and they put me on some sort of medication and that helped for a while, but still there were problems that I didn't seem to be able to sort out. A lot of it was centred around Stephen and his work and fast cars and my belief that he was not spending time with me. I wanted to be with people, yet I didn't want to be with people. And I used to feel very jealous, with a passion, of our friends. I can see now that these were all unrealistic feelings. My emotions did swing around a lot.

It is very difficult for me to pinpoint the highs and lows — except for he more dramatic ones when I was on slimming tablets. When I was given the antidepressants in the beginning they sort of helped me a little bit but I still didn't have any enthusiasm — it's very difficult to put into words. I was still tired. I can't describe how tired I felt, and I wouldn't sleep at night and things like that. I had a mania about housework at one stage. I cleaned the house every day and I didn't want people walking on the carpet. Then I had the worst low ever, in The Melbourne Clinic.

Once, when we were in Austria, I couldn't sleep very well and I used to go out in the middle of the night and walk in the snow. I would just ski really hard until about 2.00 a.m. When I didn't go out in the snow I used to sit up all night and smoke, which I suppose was very aggravating for Stephen. I don't know how he put up with it really. Once, in a fit of jealousy, I took a carving knife to him. Around that time I would often wake up in the middle of the night shaking, with my whole life going before me, like a video, in bright colour. It wasn't a dream. This happened four nights consecutively before we contacted my therapist.

The other high was in hospital... God knows why I was high. I was on another drug. They put me in hospital under observation and unbeknown to them I was allergic to whatever they gave me to quieten me down. I don't know what they were trying to get me down with, but it took a while. I seemed to cope all right after that. They are the times when I feel I've been quite off the air, for want of a better word.

I know at one time I was paranoid. I put it down to the fact that I was put in hospital by one particular medico and taken off every bit of medication that I had been on for months. I wouldn't put my worst enemy through what I went through. I shook and sweated, and I would say I went through withdrawal. I heard the telephone sixty-five times louder than it normally is in the hospital. This doctor said, 'You've been naughty, and you are going to stay here for a month without your husband — no medication, no nothing.' After that, he never came near me.

About the fourth day I started to see faces in the lino and it was pretty scary. Everybody's face in that hospital — the therapists or whoever was there — was blown up twice its size. Some of their noses were like pigs' noses, some like monkeys' and the sounds were three times the volume. I shook and sweated and had this terrible noise going on in my head at night. I felt as though someone had a whip and was belting my back. I could not lie down on that hospital bed. I was in a room with a lot of other women and I must have made an awful commotion.

Eventually they gave me a shot of something and whizzed me off somewhere. Four of them carted me off into another room where a male nurse sat and smoked with me all night, with me shaking and screaming and carrying on like a total idiot. The next morning he left me and everybody seemed to disappear and I thought, 'I've got to get out of here.'

So I packed whatever I could find and left the hospital — I didn't announce to anyone that I was leaving. Still shaking and sweating, I somehow found my way to the train then a taxi and I arrived home to my parents. My father was furious that I hadn't notified the medico because that was the right thing to do.

When Stephen eventually got me home, I really wasn't coping at all, I really was sick. In the vents of the airconditioning I could hear the voices of people I knew. I thought, 'This has got to be hell.' I never want to go through that again because I don't know whether I've got what it takes to come back again, to tell you the truth. I really believe I know what caused that. Apart from the condition itself, it was the fact that I didn't take myself off that medication — that I was taken off it by a medico. So I urge people to be very careful who they see. Sometimes you go around to different psychiatrists, seeking others' opinions because you don't quite believe what you've heard in the first place, and this can be a dangerous thing. You've got to find somebody who is a specialist, and even then trust takes a long time.

People thought I was whacko out of my mind. My husband really didn't want anything to do with me, and my children were terrified. They used to sort of walk around me. It affected my youngest daughter quite a lot and my son really didn't understand. It was quite difficult for my daughters because they're adopted. So here they were, stuck with some wacky woman who was supposed to be their mother. My elder daughter had a lot of responsibility. Her role was to be in the kitchen and the laundry and whatever. But my parents saw what was going to happen and they came and filled in. They really were a marvellous back-up. I'd come home from hospital or the clinic and I'd look at the kids and I'd think, 'My God I can't cope with you.' I didn't have any energy. I was looking for this drive that I used to have, and I didn't have it any more.

Others just thought I was a spoilt bitch. They had no idea that I was ill. I have only really got two or three friends who understand. One understands because her husband has something similar to me, and she can read me like a book. The other one is kindness itself, but really doesn't have the depth to understand the problem. One more says, 'Well, I'm sorry you've got it, but I'm glad I haven't.' Perhaps there is a little more understanding there. She came — the third one — to the clinic to see me, and I knew that it was the most uncomfortable thing for her to do. People shouldn't go under those circumstances. But everyone seems to accept me now. They've seen me at my worst, and they've seen me at my best.

I was exhausted after these episodes. Very tired. But I still couldn't sleep. It was as if there wasn't going to be any mental peace for me at all. I used to hate myself for being like I was. I didn't want to be like it. I know we all have that, but sometimes if your fantasies don't become realities there's no point in having them. So that's how I felt about it. But it wasn't long before I got to see the therapist that I'm under now, and after quite a while I began to trust him. Eventually the turning point came, and somehow I seem to have got it all together.

I have been hospitalised for depression I would say ten or twelve times, and I've been treated with medication and had occupational therapy and all that sort of thing. I guess I wasn't a terribly co-operative patient in hospital, until I came to understand that they were there to help you. I have also had quite a bit of ECT, which I don't think helped me — that's just a lay opinion. I always wondered about them counting out the tablets. I know that you go through some sort of spasm. I can remember waking up with a headache and not being able to breathe and being on a respirator, which really didn't thrill me at all. I know it's a voluntary-type situation, but I think there's lots more that can be done about it.

I didn't want to participate in group therapy. I didn't like the way people started to play psychiatrist to each other. It just wasn't my scene to be in a group. I used to make a little exclusive group of friends. I kept looking at everyone and thinking, 'Well, you've obviously got the answer to my problem', but I really didn't have any problems compared to the people I saw in there. The problem I had was probably with myself. I couldn't relate to their problems. Some of their problems were horrific and mine were nothing. And, there again, I felt at a disadvantage — rich bitch, in The Melbourne Clinic, got everything, husband comes three times a day to see her, mother trails across the other side of Melbourne to see her, everybody's pampering her. It's true, that's how they felt.

I couldn't sleep, and they don't like you not to sleep in hospitals. They like you to go to bed, and if you are asleep they find great joy in shoving a torch in your face to wake you up, so then you can't sleep. And then you get up and have coffee and annoy everybody else, or you feel like talking... that's another thing I used to do — talk a lot. That's obviously one of the symptoms of this problem of being high — I do talk very quickly.

I felt a failure. I felt that I had let my children down. I had always believed that, because my home life had been so awful, I would have a perfect life, and give my children a perfect life. My standards were unrealistically high. Therefore, when I couldn't reach all the things that I'd set my mind on, all my fantasies, I grieved, because I wanted them so badly.

Somebody once said to me, 'For Christ's sake, nobody's perfect.' I started to look around. One therapist said to me, 'You feel unhappy because your son has asthma,' and I guess in one way, yes, I resented the fact that Andrew had asthma. I was afraid that he was going to die, all the time, and I didn't trust anybody else to look after him. So I made this sort of cocoon life for myself.

Stephen used to say to me, 'Look there are people out there who have horrific lives and you've got everything.' He was trying to make me happy — materialism all the time — and it wasn't helping. All because I couldn't enjoy any of it. I resented him, I suppose, because he was normal, and he could be happy and see how beautiful the world was. He'd say, 'Look at the trees, look at the birds, look at the sea,' and I would say 'So what? It's me. I don't care about all that. I can't feel.' It was as if you were devoid of any feeling. On a hot day I'd feel cold, on a cold day I'd feel warm. It was crazy.

I attempted suicide twice. Once in earnest, and the second time I think it was attention seeking. I cut my wrists with a razor blade when Stephen was at the club, because I didn't want him out enjoying himself when I was home feeling so terrible. That frightened everybody. I used to think that I wanted to die and eventually everyone would be really sorry that they weren't kind to me. That was sympathy seeking at its best I think. I took an overdose of Valium the first time, and after that I used to just think about it. I asked my therapist to give me something. I really wanted someone else to do it for me. I'm not a brave person.

For a while there our marriage was very bad. My husband and I separated, and at one time I lived in a little flat and I couldn't cope there. Another time I totally left him, and he didn't want me back, and I stayed with my mother and father for two or three months. In the end I started to have this great desire to get back into the household. Stephen had taken the family for a holiday and while they were away I snuck back into the house and was just there when they got back.

To restore our marriage took a long time because Stephen had started to make a life for himself. He'd become slightly unbalanced himself with it all, which is understandable considering all the stress he'd been under. Stephen is really a very, very patient man, and heavily embroiled in business, which I think he threw himself into and which helped him. We feel that we've weathered a lot, yet there are some people who have weathered more. I couldn't think of anything worse than if one of the children died. But it's been a long hard struggle, not just for me but for Stephen, too. He's been very supportive.

The children can't talk about what happened to me. My elder daughter, in particular, seems to resent all the responsibility that was thrust upon her. I had a lot of trouble with my middle daughter. My son walked around me for a little while, but he is a very forgiving young man. My youngest daughter is very forgiving, too. I still feel uncomfortable at times about all this, I must say. I have tried in all ways to make up with them. It eventually worked out.

To recover and establish some order in my relationships other than my family, took, I'd say, about eighteen months. I don't have a wide variety of friends. I find that many people are too demanding. I'm too selfish for that. I get bored very easily. I'm a person who needs colossal variety in my life, and I have to make it happen. There are a couple of people I can feel are not comfortable, but that's their problem. I think I'm as good as anybody else.

I commenced lithium seven years ago. At one stage I got

smart and took myself off it slowly. My specialist did not know about this. I thought I was smart enough to take a tablet the morning I went for the blood test, so the level would be up and nobody would know. I didn't notice that I was gradually losing a lot of weight. I had a lot of energy — I would sleep but I'd get up at four in the morning and be hyperactive and do my housework or rearrange the house. I had energy so I decided that I could jog — just about killed myself, but I did it. I then started waking up at four in the morning shaking. I thought I was dying.

I couldn't drive the car, and I didn't want to go up the street to do the shopping. A girlfriend came around and she took me straight to the doctor. I had been off lithium for seventeen months, and travelled overseas without it which, of course, is not the wisest thing for anybody with my condition. So I had taken a big risk. At any rate, I was admitted and went back on lithium.

I also take Surmontil, an antidepressant, and Tegretol, to prevent fits. Occasionally I take Mogadon to help me sleep. I would like sometimes not to have to take all those damn pills at night. That is the only thing that irritates me. But I can accept myself now.

I don't feel like I can't cope any more. I don't feel tired all the time. I feel more positive. I have my doubts like everybody else. I make decisions and I think, 'My God, what have I done?' but that is a very normal human reaction. I don't feel that I have unrealistic attitudes... though sometimes my family think I have. That is where it becomes difficult: they can use it as a weapon. I won't allow it to be used. It's just... it's the difference between being dead and being alive. I think I am a much better person and far richer due to the experience that I've had. It teaches you an awful lot about humanity.

As far as creativity is concerned, I think my abilities were there before, but now my thinking process has slowed down to the point where perhaps things fit into the right boxes more easily.

People at work know about my illness. I told my boss. She has a gentleman friend who has the same problem so she doesn't worry. I've spoken to a couple of people about it, because I don't believe in keeping it shut in any more. There is a block about mental illness in society but there isn't a block in my head as much as there was.

My highlights have been various. I've always been a fairly good organiser, and I organised my son's wedding and my daughter's twenty-first — all in the one year.

I have other ambitions. Just to build the house we're building successfully, and perhaps one day to be a grandmother. I'd like to go overseas again, maybe to the Solomon Islands. I'd like to do the Whitsunday Islands. I haven't got any great big goals like going back and doing a university degree or anything like that. No, I learn from other people: the university of the world.

Anna

'It's very hard for a spouse to make the effort required to keep the family stable.'

I was an anxious child. By the time I was in my teens, both my mother and father felt that there was something wrong with me. I was already having deep fits of the blues, which didn't turn on and off over the days but went on for weeks.

I spent a lot of my time in creative pursuits such as piano, and achieved honours. I played a great deal of tennis and won trophies in this game. On the educational front, I studied and achieved a degree in social work at one of the major universities, and went on to work for many years.

In retrospect I realise what happened. I was more often depressed. When I was depressed I slowed down, I couldn't make decisions clearly, I didn't want social contact, I cried, I didn't sleep properly. It was a tremendous effort to get up and go to work or to have social activities. So there were phases in my life when I withdrew from everything, and during which I probably wasn't as efficient on the job as I could have been. I do know that in my twenties I had an unnecessary amount of absences from work due to depression.

By the time I was about twenty-four, I had what I regard now as a hypomanic attack, and I continued working while I was in this state. It shattered quite a number of people around me, and, I think, made them feel a little tenuous about their relationship with me and about my ability to do my work. It also was the first time that I really felt that something was beginning to go radically wrong. I didn't feel it during the attack because, of course, I was too euphoric. But after the attack I began to realise that I had been abnormally high, and that at other times I was abnormally low and couldn't get a grip on myself.

A number of people suggested to me that I was unbalanced. I remember in our student days, when we had to do our units on psychiatry and when manic-depressive disorder was taught, two of my friends turned to me and said, 'You know, Anna, you seem to fit that pattern very clearly.' Later on, when I had my various bouts of either depression or elation at work, there were some caring people who suggested that I go to see a psychiatrist, and in actual fact they gave me an enormous amount of support in attempting to restructure my working ability and my self-esteem. I did actually go to a psychiatrist who put me on Valium, and I went to another psychiatrist who placed me on librium, but neither of these seemed to have any long-term effect on me.

I felt very lonely with my problem. I tended at that stage still to blame my parents' long-term marital problems for my current stress. I felt worse after I had been to the psychiatrists and their treatment hadn't helped much at all. On the whole I did feel as though I was falling apart at times, and I didn't know how to get my act together again.

My first hypomanic attack at twenty-four was followed by periods of depression until I was about thirty, when I had a very severe depression, followed by some more years of relative calm — but all the time feeling an anxiety and definitely experiencing some minor episodes — until I was thirty-eight, when I had another severe depression. When I was forty I had the 'big banger' — I had a fully blown manic attack, followed by a depression.

I'll talk about my hypomanic attack first, because it is different from the manic attack. I can still remember quite clearly what happened. I was fairly high spirited at the time. I became over-talkative — I remember sitting in a staffroom at one stage and being unable to stop talking. Gradually everybody left except one person, who just sat with me while I talked, and talked, and talked. I was sexually promiscuous at the time — in fact I was after sex every day. I happened to meet a very handsome American who was out here on business, and I remember instantly moving to his hotel in the centre of the city and having days of sexual activity with him. I was elated. Within a week of having met him I bought an airline ticket to go to America with him. This behaviour continued for a short while in the USA, where I met other fellows and screwed my way around California. When the elation wore off I began to slip into a depression.

During this high I wandered into the Great Hall of the National Gallery of Victoria, and, under the splendour of the stained-glass ceiling, sat down at the Steinway grand to play Beethoven, Chopin and Fats Waller. It's the only time I've been a concert pianist. Normally I play at parties!

Now, in contrast to that, my fully blown manic attack was certainly one in which I did lose all control and insight. I became deluded and hallucinated. It was preceded a year earlier by a high episode, in which I spent some thirty to forty thousand dollars in a recording studio, thinking I had the answer to everybody's needs in music. I danced at the studio at all hours of the night and day, and constantly nagged my husband for more and more money. At the same time I hadn't realised how abnormal my behaviour was, and it didn't dawn on me how damaging it was to the family finances. I also sold our family home which threw us into disarray. We had moved into rented premises and started to reorganise our life when this fully blown manic attack occurred.

It crept up on me quietly. I didn't have any idea what was happening to me, and at first neither did my family. I remember roughly that it began with a spending spree on which I went out with a credit card and cash and bought dresses and jewellery and all sorts of things that I didn't need. I didn't want to stop myself, there was just this energy bowling me along. I was chatting up all the shopkeepers, everybody in the streets. I was everybody's great friend. Nothing could go wrong. Then I dressed up in all these clothes and I called on people and made endless social arrangements and played the life of the party generally.

But then the queer part began. I began to pull things off the walls and the shelves and out of cupboards and to give them away to people. There was this relentless drive in me to give away material possessions — I remember that I gave away a beautiful cloisonné vase, a Chinese bronze, some of my best books, my jewellery and clothing, and then at other times I threw a whole lot of these things in the rubbish bin. At that stage I was preparing to have my head shaven. I think it was only the fact that I had flights of ideas and couldn't carry out some of my projects that prevented me shaving my head.

I also believed that I was at one stage a gift from God. I had been involved in a lot of reading about ancient goddesses prior to my manic attack and I think that had an influence on my delusions. But I believed I was going to breed the great Christ child and bring him to earth again, and I found who was to be the sire of this great child. It was a Melbourne psychiatrist.

I had a preparatory bath in a friend's spa. I got out of the spa, leapt into the car and drove to the psychiatrist's home and literally just walked in and threw myself on top of him and tried to mimic intercourse. In his own inimitable way, he dealt with the situation and put me back on the road again. I sped home, still laughing and joyous, very energetic and distractable.

Later I was fearful. I thought people were after me, I was hallucinating about death, I was terrified about things like the crows in the trees, as they were foretelling of my impending death. I was very suspicious now — I wasn't jovial and sociable at all. I recall trying to make phone calls to people to tell them about what was happening, and I was so frightened that I couldn't do it in my own home. So I went down to a laundromat and hid in there and I remember hiding in an ice-cream shop and in the baker's shop.

At that stage I started drinking a great deal of red wine, I was still very argumentative, I was up in the night and wandering in the neighbourhood. I wasn't feeding my family — my husband would come home from work and find that he had all the housework and so forth to do, despite the fact that I'd been 'home all day'. He knew I was disturbed, but he didn't understand the nature and the degree or severity of the disturbance. To tell you the truth, he thought I was pretending.

By this stage, my sense of conspiracy expanded. One day I thought I had received a phone call from a friend saying that I had to go and rescue an Aboriginal woman who was being persecuted. I remember going down there, and there was a ferocious Alsatian dog that leapt all over me, all the way up the footpath, and I still persisted. I went in and organised for this woman to be removed from her home by the Aboriginal society. It was all a terrible botch and I received a message some weeks later saying that the Aboriginals never wanted to see me again. After that episode I remember driving recklessly around the roads, because by then I felt I was being followed and that I couldn't get rid of whoever was on my tail. I had to take the most circuitous routes in order to escape detention. After this I fell through the front door of a friend's house, and I lay on the floor just sobbing and sobbing. I still had no idea of what was happening to me. All I knew was this devastating fear. She managed to get me home.

On that same night I thought I had received phone calls from the deities, telling me that if I didn't get out of the house we would all be electrocuted. I remember grabbing my children and jumping into the car again, and speeding all around the neighbourhood — because I thought that various cars were following me as well, until I arrived at another friend's house. I flew through the front door and rang the police and told them that people were following me and were going to electrocute me. Of course, when the police arrived they immediately summed up the situation. I had been attending a psychiatrist at the time, and he was promptly rung. He ordered major tranquillisers — I think it was Largactil.

I had a 'bee in my bonnet' that I would be safe at my sister's place in the city, and I insisted that I be driven there. I sat in the car terrified because I thought that all the steeples were being lit up as my ceremonial procession went into the city for my impending death. We finally arrived there and my sister put me to bed, not understanding that part of the condition is that you are innately restless and distractable and confused. Of course I couldn't stay in bed. She went away and left me and I swallowed lots of Largactil. If she hadn't come in and caught me in the process, serious consequences could have taken place, because, you see, I was still deluded, I still thought I was involved in a death pact, and that I was chosen — it was a sacrifice — I was chosen to die.

While I was in her house I was very paranoid. I couldn't stand anything oriental. For some reason, I became paranoid about oriental people, and that meant anything to do with pictures or ornaments to do with an oriental flavour. So I went around the house, and I destroyed everything I could lay my hands on which had oriental eyes on it, and I turned all sorts of things to face the wall. It was then that my sister began to realise how queer I really was, but she still didn't understand what to do about it.

We came home and I set up a bonfire of all my spiritual books out in the backyard. So it went on and on and on, until finally my family stepped in. They went to the psychiatrist who was supposed to have been attending me, and roared the tripe out of him and asked him what the bloody hell was going on here. He suggested that I cool off on an ashram for a while. So I stayed on an ashram for two weeks. I certainly cooled down, I certainly stopped hallucinating and I wasn't deluded any more, but by then I was beginning to start to feel depression, and so I was hospitalised in The Melbourne Clinic. I know I was completely exhausted at the end of it. I remember at the ashram I lay on my bed for days.

If people who are suffering from this disorder, or who think they might be suffering from this disorder, can get themselves to a specialist in manic-depressive disorder they would be saving themselves a great deal of suffering. During my lifetime, I wasted years trying to find help for my condition, and I think for a person to lack quality and stability for fifteen years of their lives is a tragedy.

When I had that hypomanic bout at twenty-four, I knew afterwards that something was radically wrong with my life, and when I began to get depressed I was even more convinced that I was unstable. By that stage I had flown to London and I was feeling quite deeply depressed. I went to see a psychiatrist in one of the leading teaching hospitals. I remember I was so anxious to tell him about my sexual excesses in America that that's what we talked about mostly. And at the end of it all he told me what a dreadful person I was. Some years later, I was feeling suicidal, so I literally walked through the doors of a Melbourne psychiatric hospital and said, 'I'm sick, I need help.' Now the admitting psychiatrist took me into an office and asked me to rate my sex life on a scale of 1 to 10, had a bit of a chat with me, and then said he didn't know what they could do and sent me away. So I was very sceptical about psychiatrists. Later on, between thirty and thirty-eight, when I had moments of instability, I tried every alternative there was. I had six months of hypnosis, I went to an acupuncturist for a long time, I attended residential workshops on self-help, coping skills and self-awareness, and none of these seemed to help at all. They gave me initial bursts of elation, but that's all they achieved. Then I usually slumped back to my normal level of functioning.

I continued to bubble up and down with my instability.

But towards the end of my thirties, the ups and downs became worse. I thought, I do need to see a psychiatrist, but I will see one with a difference. So I attended a fellow who practises what they call primal therapy and I saw him for a period of almost eighteen months, during which time I had depressions, hypomania and one full-blown manic attack. The effect was so damaging and disruptive to myself and the family that they stepped in and abused this psychiatrist, and he had me referred to a specialist in manic-depressive disorders. In actual fact that's where I should have been in the first place. But even when I sought help from GPs, they didn't recognise my condition, and they didn't know who to refer me to. So, really, the message of the story is that the manic-depressive patient has to monitor him- or herself, and realise that he/she needs to see a specialist, rather than fiddling around with all these alternatives and general practitioners.

I was hospitalised when I was about forty. For the first time in a long period of time, I actually felt safe in The Melbourne Clinic. I felt as if I was in good hands. The nursing staff were wonderful, I had a provocative psychiatrist and I had comfort in my surroundings. It took some time to get used to the fact that I was in a psychiatric clinic, and that the other people in here with me were psychiatrically disturbed as well. I found it a bit upsetting at times. I remember I was sharing a room with a schizophrenic woman and with a depressed mother. But somehow or other, you acclimatise and realise that you are there for help, and that there are certain things that you need to adjust to along the road.

At that stage I was taken off all medication, because if you realise, by the time I reached the clinic, I was not manic. I was... mildly depressed. So maybe I didn't really need any of the major or minor tranquillisers. I suspect that the psychiatrist and nurses at that stage were organising this so that they could observe my behaviour in an unmedicated state. I spent two weeks there, during which I rested, indulged in group activities, socialised with the other residents, and generally pulled myself together, prior to going home. I remember, going home was the worst experience. I didn't realise how sheltered I'd been in the clinic, and I found it frightening to go home and difficult to settle down to a domestic routine or care for my children. It was some time before these things restored themselves to a normal healthy level.

I grieved about the damage done to my life, and to my family's life, and to my friends' lives, but it wasn't an instant grief. It was a growing grief, because it takes a while for you to wake up and slowly put all the details together and realise what actually happened during your attacks. When each little drop of information comes in, it's just... like a bullet, and you have to face up to the pain. I had disrupted people's lives, spent so much money, made reckless decisions, been so abominable to my family and friends, that I felt the need to be forgiven. It wasn't until someone said to me, much later, 'Forgive yourself, Anna. Forgive yourself, and start again,' that I realised how much I was grieving.

I had various levels of depressions over the years. Probably the worst one was where I was actually deluded into thinking that people were going to come and take my children away because I was an unworthy mother. I felt that there was a conspiracy of social workers and doctors who were going to organise the removal of my children. I felt filthy and had tremendous guilt and remorse. I used to lie in bed at all hours of the day, which was ironical because when I went to bed I couldn't sleep anyhow, and if I did sleep I used to wake up in anxiety. I was very, very flat. I couldn't talk to anybody very much. I found it extremely difficult if we had visitors. It was a great strain on my resources just to deal with my family, but to deal with visitors was even more... and, I know, a visible strain on me. I didn't bath myself. I remember that people commented on the fact that I hadn't even washed my hair for days. I didn't clean the house, I didn't do any washing, I didn't cook meals — my husband had to come home and do all that after work. I was not interested in any sex at all. Our sex life diminished as a result of all this. If I did get out of the house, it was just a plodding wander around the place.

There were all sorts of other symptoms but those were the worst, and again this dreadful fear pervaded the situation. I remember I used to drive my husband mad, because I used to cling to him, crying, and ask him not to go: 'Please don't leave me, please stay with me, why am I so hopeless?' — all this sort of stuff used to go on, every morning before he went to work. So that's a summary of how I experienced one of my depressions.

I have felt suicidal on a number of occasions. I know it sounds funny but I have spent time just sitting there plotting and planning with all my tablets around me, and never actually doing anything about it. The feeling is one of despair. I know at times I've actually felt that my whole family might as well be dead as well. I've tried to work out how on earth I could contrive the situation.

I was never hospitalised for depression. I was treated on an outpatient basis. In my early phases of depression, my mother, who was a nurse, looked after me lovingly and carefully, with the help of a general practitioner and antidepressants. I read as much as I could about lithium, and I decided that it was a trustworthy medication, so I have had implicit confidence in it. I take antidepressants as well to act as a buffer so that should I start to get depressed, we already have a head start. I also take stelazine, which is an anti-psychotic drug.

I would say that, ironically, the whole experience has enriched my marriage. There is a lot more honesty, trust, and warm intimacy between me and my husband now. In the earlier stages our marriage had gone through very rocky patches — in fact, I have actually run away from home, and I know he has felt like leaving on occasions, and I know at times I have told him to go. We went through a very unstable period during the time when I was most mentally fragile. It's very hard for a spouse of a manic depressive to come to terms with the effort that they have to make in order to keep the family stable, especially where children are involved. They only just get things stable, and the person has another depression, or manic attack, and so the efforts have to commence again. So there must be some loss of trust or faith and an insidious effect on their security over a long period of time. Now we seem to have built up a very harmonious relationship. We are looking forward to building even happier times together.

I'm still in the process of putting my life together again, but that's due to factors other than my manic-depressive illness. My husband's company liquidated over a year ago, and it's been very difficult for him to settle since. At the same time I discovered that, if I was to be able to work in different fields of social work, I needed extra qualifications. So, in actual fact, it's really social factors, which are nothing to do with my manic-depressive disorder, which are the big challenge at the moment.

One thing that has improved dramatically with my renewed stability is my friendships. I have networks of friends in my own neighbourhood, in my profession, where I work. Previously I was so unreliable that I'm afraid people felt that they didn't want to have prolonged contact with me. Now, I've found that I'm developing meaningful relationships which I know will last for a long time. When you are manic or depressed, people are frightened of you. They also fear their own inability to cope, and quite often they don't want to cope with it — it's too stressful. When you are stabilised and there is none of this elation or depression to intrude, things can proceed along a normal course. I'm very lucky really because two friends who saw me when I was at my worst, in either depression or mania, have stuck by me through thick or thin. However, I have to learn to discuss it openly with them. A clinical psychologist has helped me work on this. I had to overcome shame and guilt.

I think one of the most outstanding features now is that I feel that I can mostly be consistent. I still get depressed and elated, but these episodes are now modified in strength and duration.

I work as a social worker in a community health centre, and I want to be able to upgrade my standing and get into some higher administrative position. People at work don't know that I'm a manic-depressive, and I wouldn't want them to know. I feel, despite the fact that they are all in the paramedical professions, they would be unsure of me. I know they wouldn't like it because I've been involved in discussions about manic-depressive clients who've come into the centre and I didn't find the attitudes very sympathetic.

I suppose one of the highlights of my being stabilised on lithium is that I've been able to complete a musical score which has been published. Prior to going on lithium I spent an agonising amount of time trying to research and write, which was interrupted by my mood swings and which protracted the whole creative effort — so much that I felt that I really ought to give it away. In fact, on occasions I threw all my creative work in the rubbish bin.

My further ambitions now are to settle down and really enjoy the loving family life that I have, further my career in social work and publish more music.

Gregory

'I would say that lithium is the single most important ingredient in my life.'

My family is an interesting one. I have an uncle who'd be nearly sixty now. He's overseas, in the film industry, and definitely an untreated manic-depressive. He actually produces quite stunning films when he's elated. Maybe he's not so serious as to warrant treatment. I have a grandfather on the same side who is about ninety, and he has been a very uncontrollable and wild person.

In the case of my grandfather, I would say he threw fits of rage when my mother was very young and would actually beat the children. He was unmanageable at times. At other times he was very melancholic; then, at others, was enraged — more than you would expect from a normal person. He was a very difficult man to live with. I don't think that he has suffered the disease to the extent that anyone has ever done anything about it because he was born last century and they would think then that he was just a silly old so-and-so. What was the use? They were still treating patients by dunking them in cold water as late as 1905, 1910.

My uncle, on the other hand, mixes with a group of people who are pretty het-up and get pretty worked up. I've had members of the family come back and say, he's high as a kite again ... or he gets very, very depressed. That's my mother's brother. When I'm ill... when I'm manic... I consider myself to be far worse, six hundred times worse, than anyone in my family.

I feel a little bit sad because I look at the people who may have suffered — the spouses, girlfriends, boyfriends, kids. I have discussed with my present wife that there is possibly a ten-per-cent chance that we might have manic- depressive kids. I do pay strict attention to those children that are born in the family, very quietly, without discussing it much with my brother and sister. I hope their children don't become affected. However, in the long term, I think if a person wishes to be fulfilled with children, it would be silly to deny them the opportunity. With all the facilities that there are today, I don't see it as a problem. I don't see it as something where people can turn around and say, 'I'm sorry, I'm one of those, I can't have children.' It's up to the individual, and at the right time, when they feel it is something they want to do and their partner agrees.

I think in the very early stages the influences on me were probably from my mother. Her effect on me was, at that stage, greater than my father, because my father was in the Navy and he had been sent to Korea for a couple of years. He was a person who was always there in the distance, the supplier, the person who was very strong, or arrived in a uniform. A few years later, my sister came along, and then a few years after that, my younger brother. Mother doted over me and was very proud of me, and I think this set a trend until I was about fifteen or sixteen and I found myself rebelling because I felt that I should stand up on my own two feet. I was at loggerheads with my mother on many occasions in that transition of growing up. Then it became evident that there was something very wrong with me. I was about sixteen or seventeen. I couldn't cope, I failed HSC and everyone said, 'Yes, that's all right, he's just having a breakdown, pat him on the head.'

I did quite well at primary school, and when I started high school, I think I came top of the class. So I turned towards study as a way out. I think I projected myself through my hard work at school and was quite successful. However, when I got to fifth form, to everyone's shock, I failed. I went back with a lot of aggression and repeated. Then I went on to HSC and failed a couple of subjects. Five or six years ago I went back and did my whole HSC again. I need it for my work. That was my first setback, failing form five. I couldn't work out why — it upset me, threw me.

Well, actually I left HSC and I started a four-year course with a government corporation. The very first signs of illness came towards the end of the first year. I came home and I just couldn't cope. There was something wrong and I wanted to show someone that there was something wrong, so I made an attempt — to kill myself — to indicate that I could get some wires and stick them in a plug and kill myself. I did it to shock my mother to say,'Look, get off my back. There's something wrong with me.' I think a lot of people who are genuinely in trouble try to commit suicide because they are screaming out for help.

After that, I suppose I can honestly say that between the age of eighteen and twenty-three I probably had twenty jobs. I was being treated for manic-depression and I was coping with the treatment. I don't think, looking back now, that I was ready to cope with a steady job, and I worked at different places. I worked as a technician, or driving trucks and digging ditches. I did all sorts of things, and this was always a source of consternation to my family. That was a function of being ill and the extra pressure that was put on me by members of the family who said, 'Don't you forget to take those pills, you could be ill again and that would be very upsetting for all of us.' I sort of looked around and thought 'Hang on, I'm the one that got hit, I'm the one who's ill, I know it's tough for you, but do you want to swap?'

When I was about eighteen, I spoke to the local GP about my problems. I still felt lousy. More of a panic, more of a feeling of a really bad down, depression. I was lucky enough to be sent by him to a psychiatrist. He put me on a series of drugs and I can remember taking serenace — I hate that stuff. I was on the serenace but I didn't get the other drug that goes with it to stop the muscles cramping up. I can remember that stuck out in my mind, that horrific effect. I went home for two weeks. It was my first two weeks home, and of course I was having problems. So I spent nine months on things like counselling, drugs, and a series of shock treatments. It actually helps you, because you can forget certain patches of things and it's supposed to align everything. When I came out, I relapsed and went in again. So, my psychiatrist said to me, 'We are going to try this lithium carbonate.' I started on the stuff, and did very well. A period of time, I think five years, went by before there were any more problems. That period of time was when I became involved with my previous wife, got married. Things were quite stable in that time. I was twenty-two by then. Well, it was an oasis, if you know what I mean.

I can remember in the early stages that my father would come in to me — I'd be in bed, shaking all over and not coping with anything — and he would just hold my shoulders. He would just put his arms on me so I'd stop shaking and it felt really good. My father was very confused. He couldn't understand why his big son — Number One, first born son — had packed it in. He would always come in and hold me and look at me and he would say, 'We are going to beat this.' I was the wimp son who couldn't cope, and I think that idea played merry hell with me when I was young.

I've had a few episodes in my life, at least two depressions and two manias, with a five-year gap. One side- effect of my treatment was a kidney scare four or five years after I was married. It was indicated to people that lithium could harm kidneys, and the doctors did everything they could to help. My doctor said he'd like me to taper down my lithium carbonate. I think I lasted eighteen months on nothing. Then my behaviour changed, and I knew something was wrong and my first wife argued with me about it. I had been wandering South Australia. After twelve months over there I came back to Melbourne, bought a home and got settled in, and then my whole life came undone.

I think I collapsed in the bedroom of my own home, I just stood up and fell down, and I felt... yuk, all over. I think that there were a lot of pressures on me at the time. I'd just bought a home, my parents were bringing my grandparents out, and they'd bought a home around the corner, and I was angry. I had an argument with my parents about moving to within half a mile of me. I was not under any treatment, and I was trying as best I could to cope, but I just couldn't — my body couldn't cope. I started seeing things, I'd look at something and it would go sideways. I started to imagine that my life was getting out of hand. I had delusions about God and Jesus Christ. That's when I ultimately ended up in the back of a divvy van.

I owe a great debt to the Victoria Police. They are a marvellous bunch of guys. They try very, very hard and they get the rough end of the deal. If you are out there running around on the freeway, they've got to get you and put you in a van and take you out to Larundel. I ran away from the hospital once, and they put a thing on my leg so I couldn't walk properly, so I'd slow down. I went there for the first time and then, two years later, went there again, under the most horrific circumstances of being tracked down by police. I was herded like an animal. From my point of view, being a manic-depressive, I felt like I was at the end of the earth. It was so humiliating.

I had been difficult to catch and violent. It took five policemen to escort me to hospital. I had spoken of giving my house away, and gave money to a patient while at the doctor's. I could not concentrate due to the rapid flow of ideas in my mind. I was also very talkative.

So you go there and you expect this horrible dungeon of horrors, and yet they're human, real, and caring. You start out in solitary confinement and... I never stayed there very long, but long enough to see that it's a catchment area, it's a place where you calm down a bit; and respond to medication.

The second time it happened, I had stopped my lithium. With my past history it was a silly thing to do. I became very over-active. I had been admitted to The Melbourne Clinic and attempted to abscond several times. I ran around the car park until I was exhausted, giving my psychiatrist a couple of frightening bear hugs on the way past. I had to be transferred to Larundel for further restraint.

I was very high, uninhibited, talking a great deal, kissing the doctor, and apparently had little insight. I believed myself to be persecuted by a work mate, and even thought he was a rapist.

The occasions of becoming ill are probably the most frightening experiences that I've ever gone through. You try to bluff it out, through your life. You say you're a big strong man and not going to be frightened of anything. But a manic attack is a very frightening experience. It is certainly frightening for people around you, and your loved ones whom you care for. They have to make decisions, bring in doctors and police, and they feel terribly responsible that they have done you harm. It's the best thing they can do to try and contain you until you can get medication and calm down.

Most of my attacks have involved wandering aimlessly around. On one occasion they found me on the Princes Highway out past Dandenong in the centre of the freeway, walking along in the bushes in the middle. I was unable to give any real reason why I was there.

With these attacks — the two bad ones, and four overall — I inevitably ended up in Larundel. Frightening as that place can appear to some people, it was terrific for me because I knew that it was all over.

I think people have got the wrong idea about manic attacks. They get this idea that we are going to go out there and kill somebody. I've never ever had any desire to destroy or hurt anybody. It's only an elated feeling... I suppose it's like breathing helium or too much oxygen or something. There's an old saying that when you cross a desert and you've got a thirst you wouldn't swap it with anyone because it's going to feel so good when you quench it. I think that's the positive way of looking at it. You don't know you are ill and when someone tracks you down and puts you in a paddy wagon, that first injection will knock you out and bring you back to earth.

You become possessed with the idea that you have a goal to achieve. You have to get there, but you are not quite sure why you have to get there, or if somebody's told you you've got something special to do or whatever, you have this strange feeling that you've really got to go. You don't have a lot of insight at the time.

I can remember people coming towards me — and they must have been ordinary people — and they looked like they were out of the Spastic Society, since their faces were all distorted. So my ability to see a normal person was obviously all twisted. I also remember getting on a train at Box Hill station. The train seemed to swap tracks, and I couldn't work out which way to get out of the train. I couldn't get off it, and I just hung on until it stopped at a station and I got out what I thought was the right door. The effect of the attack on me was... frightening.

I don't think I ever physically accosted anyone. I can remember having a fight with my father when I was manic. He took a lovely right hook swing — he was a boxer in the Navy — and he split my lip. He was trying to pin me down, and I had a go at him and shouted. After that I had a shouting match in the street, and of course all the neighbours wondered what was going on, but I think he was protecting the home. He wouldn't let me in the house, because he knew how much stress I was putting on my mother.

A classic statement that my wife made after my illness and after the divorce was that she felt that it would have been easier for her if I'd died in hospital. I understood that she had gone through a terrible time. Her mother came over and stayed with her, helped her, instructed her, and when I came home from hospital the message was clear that she wished to leave. She left. I said, 'Take whatever you want,' so she took everything. After eight weeks in hospital, I came out very groggy, shaky as all hell. I went down the road with my father and we unlocked the house and walked in. I was emotionally upset because of the fact that the marriage was over. The house was empty, the vegetable garden was dead, and the past was gone, not because of anyone's fault. I can feel for my wife. I can say, 'Yes, it must have been dreadful.' It must have been hard to be married to someone for four or five years and have them go through an episode, just one episode. I sympathise, but I'll say this much: I have met women who are married to men in wheelchairs, and they cope.

I think the only regrettable thing about manic- depression, especially in my case, is that people don't want to talk about it. There is no room for discussion, we must cover it up. My mother, on one occasion, insisted that I take half a pill more, because she felt more of it would shut me up. I went through an horrific week and a half, or two weeks, and said, 'There you are, you're wrong.' It's sad that you can't go into the tearoom at work and sit down and discuss it. You can't really. You would like to. You feel that it would be nice. What a wonderful society it would be where you could sit down and discuss it freely.

After one attack, I started out with exactly $47 in the bank, I had no job, and I rented a caravan in mum and dad's backyard. I refused to take it for free. I said I wanted to pay... but I only had a few shirts and bits and pieces. I got enough money together and rented a place. All I know is that I got sick, so I started again.

I had a manic attack, and went to Larundel — this was the fourth one, the last one. So I still stuck to my guns when I came out and I moved in really close to work. Mother said, 'You'll never find anywhere there. You won't succeed, you haven't got anything,' but while she was saying that (I think she was stirring me up) she was lending me table cloths and forks and knives.

You keep going home and you think, 'I don't believe this has happened'. You don't forget the shock of the attack, and the fact that you're a person who is divorced. Throw the manic attacks away and say look at the person from the point of view of the tremendous upheaval of losing someone and all the turmoil that goes with that.

So, there I am, sitting with the two things on the mantel shelf looking at me. I think one of the best things I ever did was when I picked up my kit bag, and went back to play football. I walked back to my old club and they'd gone, and another club was there. They looked at me and said, 'You're six foot. Do you play well in the forward pocket?' I said, 'Oh yeah.' So I started to train, and I started to take out my aggression or my hurt on a Sherrin football. I did not go out on the field and punch people in the head or physically hurt people. I tackled and tackled hard, but I think I was punishing myself. I think I was saying, 'You naughty person, you're a manic-depressive, you've ruined your life.' I got out on the football field and I ran. I think I played some of the best games of my life. The coach would say, 'There he goes again.' Not as high as a kite, just a normal person — footy jumper on, mud all over me, falling over, picking up the ball, kicking it, working with a team.

Making friendships began again. I had a young lady who worked with us. She missed a few days through illness and was told that she had to make up the time. It was winter at the time and one of the senior chaps said, 'I'll give you a lift home.' One night at six o'clock, I was going home late and I saw her. I said, 'What are you doing?' She said she had to catch a bus. I said, 'You're not going to walk four hundred metres from this place in the dark. I'll take you home. I'll see a senior officer about it tomorrow.'

I dropped her off, and the other chap would drop her off, too. We worked out a routine. Not very far away her parents ran a take-away restaurant. One day she said, 'Why don't you come in and meet my folks?' This was someone saying thank you for giving me a lift. I got a free pizza, I sat down, I spoke to the people. I've know them for five or six years. They are the greatest friends I've got. I used to go down there after work, and I would wash up and do the washing. They were Spanish, and there were lots of other people who would come in and talk. All the families, and that whole community of people, I still know. Those people, being very hard-working and versatile, opened a bridal shop. I was lucky to have them design my second wife's wedding dress for her wedding day. I owe them a great deal because I wasn't the most easy person to get on with.

When I got sick I had been working for twelve months to eighteen months in my present job. I've been there for nine years, and I've worked my way up. I work in the scientific profession. I'm a technical officer, in a medical and dental laboratory. Having been good with my hands, and pretty adept with my brain, I started off as just a technical assistant, Grade 1, ages ago. Anybody who works for the Government has to be patient. I think the quality you most need in this profession is to be well ordered. If you want to bust a great big block of sticks, right, you don't try and bust the sticks, you break one at a time, and you get through it. So a calm, ordered mind, organisation and the 'bundle of sticks' principle are my chief qualities in my role.

The Government requires, for superannuation purposes, that the medical officer and the senior officer know that I suffer manic-depression. But there are members of staff who've been there long enough to remember, or witness one of my last attacks. They saw me ill. We've got one or two people who have come to us who have had these so-called nervous breakdowns. They've come from top management back down to our level, so I don't generally sit with them and chat with them about it, because it might upset them. But the thing is, it's not something I wear on my sleeve.

I commenced lithium in 1971. I also take a very small amount of thyroxine because of one of the slight side-effects. After quite a few years — not in everybody but in a few people — the pituitary gland doesn't function so well, so we feed it 50 mg of thyroxine. This produces a slight swelling in the neck. I'm not going to jump up and down and say lithium is the greatest thing on the earth, but I would say coolly and calmly that it is the single most important ingredient in my life. Priadel, which I've taken for the last seven years, has been really good. It has brought about enormous stability for me. You can see it in my history, if you put the two together. It is of great clinical relevance.

My psychiatrist is the other essential ingredient for my health. The main point about psychiatrists is that they have to study medicine first. They are qualified physicians, and some of these guys specialise in all sorts of things. They work phenomenal hours, they are incredibly dedicated people, and the pressure that they are under because of the types of people must be great. My psychiatrist talks frankly to me and he exudes a certain amount of calm and a consistency. I do feel that my relationship with him is one of really good friends; we are two people who work towards the one aim. You need that link, because without it you can't administer to yourself and you shouldn't try. The biggest problem people have is accepting that there is something wrong. Once you've decided yes, there is a problem, the next thing is to say, I've got to do something about it, and go along to a specialist. I must admit there is a certain about of trepidation about lithium when it comes to levels and readings, but I more or less look at it as a necessity. The psychiatrist will examine you sometimes with a stethoscope and take your blood pressure — so I don't really regard it as any more of a hassle than to go to a GP. It should be promoted as such. I've met people who are terrified of psychiatrists.

Now? Well, I'm very happy. I think that I have equipped myself, from a personal point of view, with enough of the skills and enough of the learnt lessons, sometimes the hard way, to first of all cope with life and life's everyday problems. I would describe myself as someone who is travelling in a certain direction, with my career and my family. I have a good future. I honestly can sit down and say, well, if you can get that far, surely you can get a bit further down the track. But I try very hard not to look too far into the future, or have too grand an idea of what I can do. I think I'm happy because I'm satisfied that I've got the right combination and that I'm doing the right things, and with the help of my doctors and friends, and especially my wife, and people like that, I think that that's more than I ever could have wished for.

My main task at the moment is bringing up a seven-year-old boy. That boy keeps me going; he's fantastic. He wanted to buy me a Father's Day present. I said to him, 'Why do you want to buy me a Father's Day present, because I'm not really your dad?' and he said, 'Well, you're almost my dad.' Those are the things, the million-dollar statements. You sit there and pat him on the head, and to him it's just one sentence in another million sentences.

We have worked very hard, my wife and I, to provide him with a home. We've bought a Victorian terrace house; it's nothing flash but it's down in Middle Park and its a little old-fashioned hundred-year-old cottage. We wouldn't swap it for the world. We go fishing and have picnics together. Josie's getting back a little bit of what she missed out on. I'm getting a little bit back, and I sit there sometimes and I think... Once when Winston Churchill was at school he was asked 'What would you do when everything is nearly lost?' He said, 'There are only nine words: never give in, never give in, never give in.' I'm going to paint that on my wall.

The greatest highlight in my life was to marry my second

wife. But I suppose one of the others was to complete that first HSC subject just to prove to myself that I wasn't a dodo brain. Other things would be the overall effect on the families involved, and my wife's ex-husband accepting the fact that Tim, her son, has a right to be loved and to be cared for, nicely balanced, with one grandma on his side, and one grandpa on my side. I think that's been a very, very tough struggle, but that is a highlight. I think my wife is included because she tried very hard. Career-wise, I know there's a chance for advancement coming up in the future and I would be silly not to aspire to that position after nine years in the department.

I seek for my family and my wife and I just to drift away from the storm a bit, sit in the calm and bask.

5

COMMON QUESTIONS

A number of questions come up repeatedly in conversations between sufferers of mood disorder and their psychiatrists or therapists. We have included a representative sample here.

Question:
Will I ever have manic or depressive attacks now I am taking lithium?

Answer:
You might, but the possibility is significantly reduced. Of the eight people whose stories feature in this book only one has had an attack since lithium treatment, and they had been taking lithium for seven to fifteen years. The available data suggests that three out of four people will never have significant mania or depression again.

However, if an attack does occur, your prophylactic lithium therapy will probably make it less severe and shorter in duration, and not requiring hospitalisation. If you monitor yourself, or ask someone close to you to do this, you can seek help early and thus further reduce the severity of the attack.

Question
Will I ever be able to stop taking lithium?

Answer:
This is rather like asking 'Will I always have this disease?'

The disorder affects one for life; and many people, if untreated, have an increasing number of attacks as they age. For most people on lithium therapy the risks of ceasing it are too great. If you recall the last attack you experienced, it will remind you of the risks. It is also difficult to predict when attacks will occur, and people who have jobs, families, and social lives to consider cannot afford the risk of being without lithium. There are, however, some people who, because their illness develops slowly and predictably, can be treated only after the beginning of an episode, and others whose attacks occur at a particular time of the year and therefore need to take lithium for that period only.

Question:
Why would one want to stop taking lithium?

Answer:
Perhaps because of rebellion, fear of toxicity, wanting more creative energy, feeling unrealistically that you are now cured, or missing manic elation — these are some of the reasons people cease lithium therapy. All these issues are dealt with under various other questions in this chapter.

Question:
Why should I take a toxic drug?

Answer:
Relatively few sufferers are affected by toxicity, and these can be quickly and effectively treated by doctors. Unfortunately there is often a narrow margin between the effective treatment dose and one high enough to produce troublesome side-effects and the risk of poisoning. Nonetheless there is no treatment of bipolar mood disorder that is more potent or successful than lithium. As already mentioned in this book, the advantages of taking the drug far outweigh the disadvantages for the vast majority of sufferers.

To allay fears, make sure you and your family know the signs of impending lithium poisoning. The psychiatrist should be contacted if even one of these signs appears. A blood test will be taken to determine serum lithium concentration, and the dosage altered depending on the results.

A person with impending lithium poisoning should also drink copious quantities of water. Depending on the severity of symptoms, you may be treated as an outpatient, or be admitted to hospital. For details on lithium poisoning see Appendix II.

Question:
Could this problem have existed in a mild undiagnosed form earlier in my life?

Answer:
A search of the histories of sufferers reveals that many people have experienced symptoms commencing in the teenage years or even earlier. The presence of mood disorder may not have been diagnosed due to reluctance to seek help, confusion with 'normal' adolescent turmoil, infrequency of episodes, moving to another locality, change in doctors and so forth. If families seek help early on, the prospects for study, career and relationships are not so diminished. The self-esteem of a sufferer also needs consideration. The longer a person struggles alone, the greater the possible damage to their self-esteem or morale.

Inevitably the question arises as to whether sufferers should observe their children for symptoms. While your children might not experience the disorder, and undue observation or questioning might upset them, being alert to the possibility can ensure that help is obtained early. Teenagers with mood disorder can present with behavioural problems, school failure, 'dropping out', and drug addiction, including alcoholism. It is best to acquaint yourself with the symptoms described in this book, and seek help if you are concerned. Alternatively, to keep matters in perspective, consult a psychiatrist before approaching the young adult.

Question:
I am upset at being labelled a sufferer of bipolar mood disorder. What can I do?

Answer:
There is a saying that 'labels are for jam jars, not for people'. However, until an accurate diagnosis of any illness is made, no effective treatment can be prescribed for the short or long term. Sufferers of diabetes or arthritis, for example, are also faced with accepting a diagnosis, or label.

The underlying reasons for your feelings might be having a psychiatric condition, the manner in which you have been handled, the fact that you need to take drugs, loss of your perceived self, or feeling that you have let yourself down.

You can choose to work on your responses to this labelling with a psychiatrist, a clinical psychologist, or another psychotherapist. Your feelings need to be constructively managed rather than allowed to become anti-social or to turn inwards. You need to confront the pain, anger, loss and self-loathing. If it is a struggle to accept, seek help. You can gain a great deal of support from working through the issues of self-acceptance and self-love. Paradoxically, in expressing your vulnerability you can find your strengths.

You are, despite being diagnosed as suffering from bipolar mood disorder, a unique person with needs, desires, dreams, successes or failures, and creativity. You will develop a pathway in life where you can realise some of your ambitions. A new quality of stability may characterise relationships as the effects of lithium treatment take hold. In time you will re-focus on yourself as a person, not a diagnostic category.

Question:
Highs should be pleasurable. Why do I become suspicious and fearful?

Answer:
Not all people suffering mania are happy. A certain number develop delusions and hallucinations which are frightening. Those experiencing hypomania often report having had a wonderfully high episode which they would have liked to last for ever. But some of these go 'over the top' and become psychotic, which is a fearful experience. In interviews included in this book, you will be able to determine who was paranoid (or suspicious) and who was not. If you read carefully you will notice that suspicions invade the suffering of depression as well.

Some people have a personality which is more prone to mistrust and suspicion, and these people may have more of these features during their manic or depressive attacks.

We must remember that the sufferer implicitly believes the truth of these suspicions and acts upon them, causing a great deal of damage in their lives. The poem at the beginning of this book shows guilt-ridden suspicions about the children being taken away, a fear characteristic of the depressive phase. The manic phase in the poem depicts a plot to have relations with gods, a delusion which involves suspicion.

A person with paranoid (suspicious) tendencies may have difficulty in thinking realistically even when well. This is the feature of the personality, not the disorder. Paranoia can be easily triggered in these people, and usually consists of suspicions about what people are saying, imagining plots against them, seeing rejection where there is none, and fear of authority figures.

It can be difficult to tease out what is really occurring and what is imagined, and this results in a great deal of anxiety and stress for the person. If the paranoid person has insight it may be even more stressful because they recognise suspicious thoughts as being irrational but cannot stop them.

Because of this, relationships can be harmed, jobs lost and self-esteem reduced. It is vital to seek help for this. Your psychiatrist will know what paranoid tendencies you have, and will negotiate with you regarding an appropriate treatment. Medication can help, and so can special techniques to facilitate thinking and rational responses, guided by clinical psychologists who practise cognitive behavioural therapy.

Question:
Why are women more likely to suffer mood disorder than are men?

Answer:
Statistically, women are twice as likely as men to suffer major depression and twice as likely to attempt suicide. There might be a number of reasons for this.

Much feminist literature suggests that chronic oppression is a significant cause. Women suffering unstable relationships, chronic socio-economic problems, abuse or trauma seem more vulnerable to mood swings. There is also evidence that many women who relinquish their children at birth will suffer intermittent major depression. Oppression often causes loss of self-worth, guilt and loss of identity, resulting in powerlessness, helplessness and suppressed rage. These coincide with some of the warning signs of major depression.

Question:
How can I make sure I don't meet with further oppression in the psychiatric situation?

Answer:
It is true, regrettably, that some women feel misunderstood by their male psychiatrist because of his different world view. This can compound the feelings of helplessness that made treatment necessary in the first place. Women should shop around, and

listen to the recommendations of others, to find a therapist who genuinely understands women's issues.

Question:
Do the public and private health systems offer the same opportunities for treatment and management of mood disorder?

Answer:
Treatment of mood disorder and care of sufferers is similar throughout all clinics and hospitals in Australia. All treatments described in this book are provided by both, with the exception of psychotherapy, which might be less accessible in public hospitals than in private clinics. However, some psychologists, social workers and nurses in the public system help patients develop skills for coping, while occupational therapists assist in social skills training, anger management and occupational skills.

Question:
Why was I humiliated by being certified?

Answer:
Certification means you are detained for a period of time, having been assessed by a psychiatrist as being seriously ill and requiring inpatient treatment, in spite of your belief to the contrary. This is aimed to protect you as well as your loved ones and/or colleagues. It assures you of appropriate treatment and response.

However, manic patients typically do not enjoy being crossed, reject the notion that they are ill and need treatment, are very restless, often physically overpowering and try to attain power in all situations. If the person is deluded and hallucinating, suffering from flight of ideas and paranoia, then they do not respond to reasoning. They are a danger to themselves and threatening to those around them, and need urgent medical treatment.

There seems to be no truly humane way of dealing with an unmanageable person, given the trauma of being manhandled by up to five police, locked in a van after a struggle, certified, taken to a strange hospital and injected with tranquillisers. The experience can take some time to recede in the manic person's mind.

It is not surprising that you feel humiliated by having been certified. But, to put it in perspective, you might like to spare a thought for the sufferers who wish they had been caught at the height of their psychotic mania, certified and hospitalised. The damage they created in all aspects of their lives left them with great remorse and took several years to repair.

Question:
What will happen to my mental ability?

Answer:
Mental abilities are not impaired by mood disorder, unlike some types of schizophrenia which can cause gradual deterioration. Despite this fact, many sufferers take time to adjust to the absence of manic highs, and might therefore, at times, feel as though their mental abilities are diminished.

Also, initially, when taking the medication required for mania or depression, you might experience side-effects which make you think you have lost some mental abilities. Poor concentration, lack of alertness, difficulties in making decisions, distractability, or apathy might all give you cause for concern. Some people complain that lithium reduces their creativity, but this is variable. Creativity is dealt with under another question.

If, however, you are stabilised on lithium, any signs of marked apathy, lowered concentration, sleepiness or indistinct speech might denote impending toxicity.

Memory might occasionally be impaired due to depression, changes in activity of the thyroid gland, or the lithium dose itself. All of these problems can be corrected.

Sometimes established personality characteristics are confused with greater or lesser mental ability. Some people are troubled by preoccupations and compulsions, others are paranoid or might be anti-social or destructive in relationships. If necessary, you can discuss with your psychiatrist any troublesome aspects of your personality and the steps you might take to remedy them.

Question
Can I pass this on to my children?

Answer:
Although some people with bipolar disorder have no family history of mood swings, most sufferers can identify relatives with a history very suggestive of mania and/or depression.

Overall the incidence of bipolar mood disorder in immediate relatives (parents, siblings, children) is about fifteen per cent, or slightly less than one in seven. For identical twins, if one twin has the disorder, there is a seventy-per-cent chance of the other twin developing it, whether or not they are raised in the same family.

The fact that thirty per cent of identical twins — that is, people with identical genes — do not become victims shows that it is not just faulty genes that decide whether or not a person develops bipolar mood disorder. Life experiences must also be a factor.

Although, statistically speaking, the chance of one of your children having the disorder is about one in seven (or greater if your spouse also carries the gene), the genetic dice might turn up a favourable result (no children with bipolar disorder) or a bad one (all with it). Looking on the bright side, the fact that you have been correctly diagnosed will make life easier for any of your children with the faulty gene because earlier diagnosis is likely.

Question:
What can I expect from my psychiatrist?

Answer:
A psychiatrist is a physician who monitors your health and prescribes medication, adjusting it as necessary. He or she also possesses skills in psychiatric diagnosis, physical illness, personality assessment and counselling, plus knowledge about social issues affected by health problems. With such skills a psychiatrist is an effective counsellor, despite the fact that a session might just seem like a chat.

If you have protracted and deep-seated problems, your psychiatrist might assess that more time-consuming therapies are necessary and therefore refer you to someone who specialises in these, such as a psychiatrist or psychologist who is specially trained in what is known as psychotherapy. If you have a low income, a private clinical psychologist might be too costly for you. Treatment without charge is available at public hospitals and community health and psychiatric centres, as well as from some non-profit voluntary counselling services associated with religious and lay organisations.

Question:
Will I ever be creative again?

Answer:
A swing into the blues, personal problems, fatigue or stress can have an inhibiting influence on creativity in the lives of anyone, not only sufferers of bipolar mood disorder. Creativity also comes in waves, with peaks and troughs, which again is something all people experience, and possibly need to come to terms with.

During mania one can, due to extreme distraction and disorganisation, overestimate the value of one's creative efforts. Depression, on the other hand, brings its own misery and lack of productivity. The sense of stability that you stand to gain from taking lithium is reassuring compared with this roller-coaster effect.

Creativity can be reduced by lithium, but the majority of creative people find that the effect is minimal and their usual high-quality output can be achieved. Individuals are creative despite their disorder, not because of it. The creativity is inherent in the personality, and after a phase of mania or depression, can return with full force.

Of course, not all sufferers of bipolar mood disorder are highly creative, and not all creative people are sufferers. However, mood swings and alcoholism, suicide and drug taking have seemed to plague creative people in particular throughout history. While lithium reduces or modifies these behaviours, creativity persists.

Business people often fear a reduction in their capacity to create new ideas, make decisions, interact effectively, and maintain the requisite pace if they take lithium. Some, monitored carefully by the psychiatrist, take lithium and other drugs only when they sense an approaching attack of mania or depression. Others are on a dose of the drug which is so low that it might not be sufficient to protect them from an attack.

Creative people tend to be eccentric, erratic, out of the ordinary and, in particular, more prone to emotional problems than the general population. In order to allow creativity to flow and produce results, these people might well benefit from therapies that aim to help with problem-solving, such as those described in the previous chapter.

Creativity is probably a delicate special balance of talent, discipline and inherited chemical energy. It flourishes in the right environmental conditions. When seeking a change in job, contacts, friends or clubs, you could perhaps assess whether they are stimulating enough to nurture your creativity.

Whenever possible, psychiatrists carefully evaluate patients' adaptation to chronic, recurrent mood disorder, especially those who continue to earn income during mild hypomanic phases. If the high produces success and wellbeing without serious annoyance to others, the psychiatrist will determine whether or not it is therapeutically expedient to leave it alone.

Some creative people become so accommodated to their mild highs and lows that they consider these episodes as basic facets of their personalities and really do not want to change them. If you are one such person, you might care to raise the matter of creativity with your doctor.

Question:
Will I work again?

Answer:
If you wish to, with some possible changes. You might glean some helpful tips from the following list of methods that other sufferers have used to remain in or return to the workforce.

- Re-arrange your curriculum vitae to cover gaps in employment due to illness.
- Accept humble work in order to begin again.
- Reconsider options and start a course to retrain in another career.
- Take part-time work in lieu of full-time, supplemented w creative work.
- Re-assess your abilities and downgrade jobs if unable to cope with pressure.
- Accept a position under supervision until you have developed confidence and expertise again.
- Take refresher courses in your chosen field.
- Seek psychological counselling for modification of worrying problems in your area of work, and apply prescribed strategies on the job.

Question:
What if I lose my job or am discriminated against due to my condition?

Answer:
If you exhibit florid symptoms of mania or are dysfunctional

due to depression, an employer might well dismiss you. There is a stigma attached to psychiatric disorder and, unfortunately, once trust has been lost, people might not wish to persevere with you. Nor are employers or staff particularly interested in the possibility of you becoming well, even if you are having psychiatric help.

You might have to accept dismissal, and start again when you are well, taking care to stay on your medication and seeing your psychiatrist regularly.

Depending on the circumstances, your psychiatrist might act as an advocate for you, developing some conciliatory strategies. Some people can themselves negotiate with their employers and might be accepted, with or without special conditions. Those dealing with more subtle problems — such as derision, difficulty in gaining responsibility, harassment, unrealistic guidelines, and so on — might well have a case for an appeal. Equal Opportunity Commissions and industrial relations tribunals deal with these matters and with unfair dismissal. Having assessed your problems, they will negotiate with employers and staff for a reconciliation or for compensation. They also provide information on your rights as an employee with an illness. Nowadays, with widespread protection of people who are suffering from physical diseases or handicaps, there is fertile ground for those with psychiatric problems to seek support. It takes courage and patience, and one has to be prepared to sit in conciliation meetings and take the possible consequences of such actions.

However, depending on how you feel about your future career, you might, under some circumstances, be better advised to withdraw gracefully and start again elsewhere.

Question:
How can I stop any employer finding out about my disorder?

Answer:
Regrettably, because discrimination against patients with psychiatric disorder is still prevalent, it is prudent to take reasonable precautions to prevent your disorder becoming known in the workplace. We suggest the following means of achieving this:

- Be sure to take your prescribed medication, and see your psychiatrist as often as requested.
- If possible, take your medication at home. If you really need

to take it at work, keep it concealed and swallow it in privacy.

- Don't talk with colleagues about your symptoms and problems. Find an external counsellor with whom to discuss your health.
- Take sick leave when unwell.
- Learn to know your limitations and stay clear of demands which are too taxing.
- If necessary, develop pursuits that give you a basis for general communication with colleagues — sport, art, music. This steers the subject away from the personal.
- Wear long sleeves on the day of your lithium blood test in order to conceal the mark left by the needle.
- Avoid excessive alcohol — it might make you babble!

Appendix I

MEDICATIONS COMMONLY PRESCRIBED

Antidepressants

Tricyclics

amitriptyline
clomipramine
desipramine
dothiepin
doxepin
imipramine
nortriptyline
trimipramine

Monoamine Oxidase Inhibitors (MAOIs)

phenelzine
tranylcypromine

Reversible MAOIs

moclobemide

Other Antidepressants

mianserin
fluoxetine

Antipsychotics

chlorpromazine
fluphenazine
haloperidol
pericyazine

pimozide
thioridazine
thiothixene
trifluoperazine

Mood Stabilisers

carbamazepine
lithium carbonate
sodium valproate

Benzodiazepines

alprazolam
bromazepam
diazepam
flunitrazepam
lorazepam
nitrazepam
oxazepam
temazepam

FURTHER INFORMATION ON LITHIUM

The subject of lithium treatment is covered broadly in Chapter 4 of this book. The purpose of this appendix is to provide further detailed technical information on this medication.

What Is Lithium?

Lithium is a naturally occurring substance — the lightest known metal. It is closely related to the well-known substances sodium (which, as sodium chloride, is common salt) and potassium. No other mineral is as widely used, or as important as a specific mineral medical treatment. In fact, more articles are published in scientific journals on the subject of lithium than on any other medication.

Although small amounts of lithium are normally found in the body, it does not have a major role in cell metabolism or function, though its close relatives, sodium and potassium, are very important.

The level of lithium required for effective treatment of mood disorder is a thousand times greater than the level normally found in the body. Mood disorder is not, as some people mistakenly believe, caused by deficiency of lithium, any more than rheumatoid arthritis, which is sometimes treated with gold, is caused by a deficiency of gold.

Sodium and potassium are involved in producing the energy in cells which enables them to carry out their function, maintaining the body's activities and, indeed, life itself. Lithium appears to exert its beneficial effect by stabilising the process which produces energy within the cell.

How Does Lithium Work?

Lithium is taken in tablet form, as the salt lithium carbonate. The vast majority of prescriptions in Australia are for Lithicarb (250 mg) or Priadel (400 mg) which is a slow-release form.

Lithium takes time to produce a therapeutic effect. When given to a patient suffering from an episode of mania the benefit might not be observable for five to ten days (during which phenothiazines are given). Its influence in preventing the recurrence of mood swings is not maximal in many patients until they have been taking it for about a year.

For some unknown reason patients in the manic phase are often able to tolerate high doses of lithium (doses which would cause toxic symptoms if continued after the episode has settled).

The average dose required to maintain a level of lithium in the blood (which actually affects the level in the rest of the body) is about 1200 mg per day. The major factor which determines the dose is the level of kidney function. Young people might require up to 2400 mg of lithium carbonate per day, whereas elderly patients, whose kidneys are less efficient, might need only 250 to 400 mg per day.

Because lithium is potentially toxic, it is usually given in at least two doses per day, approximately twelve hours apart, to reduce the peak levels in the blood. Dividing the daily dose into three or four different medication times would reduce the peak levels even more, but unfortunately people tend to forget medication when it is prescribed to be taken more often than at morning and night, and a regular lithium intake is vital if blood levels are to remain within therapeutic limits — that is, between the lowest level which is effective and the level at which toxic symptoms can occur.

Blood tests to measure the level of lithium in the body are carried out at decreasing frequency as the level stabilises. Although they might need to be measured twice a week at the beginning of treatment, tests at two- to three-monthly intervals are the norm for long-term therapy, unless illness, the introduction of other medications or a change in dose indicates that earlier testing is advisable.

Side-effects

As with most powerful medications, lithium can have some side-effects, but most patients feel these are minor compared with the benefits of a stable mood and increased well-being.

The most common side-effects are:

- **Tremor:** A slight shakiness in the fingers might affect writing. This might be most obvious a certain number of hours after you take the medication, and you might be able to avoid writing at this time.
- **Thirst:** Lithium carbonate is like ordinary salt and causes thirstiness but it does not increase blood pressure as salt does. Patients taking lithium must quench their thirst. This is expecially important in hot weather, and particularly for older people, as dehydration increases the concentration of lithium in the blood. (Other antidepressant or anti-manic drugs might cause a dry mouth, rather than thirst. Patients can alleviate dryness by sucking low-calorie lollies or jubes.)
- **Passing more urine:** Partly because of increased intake of fluids, and partly because lithium reduces the ability of your kidneys to concentrate urine, you will urinate more often. This problem rarely becomes severe, but if it does, inform your doctor. Under these circumstances you might have to stop taking lithium, but this is most unusual. Very rarely, permanent reduction of function and changes to the structure of the kidneys might occur. Your doctor will check your kidney function every six to twelve months.
- **Weight gain:** This is a problem for many people taking lithium. It is partly a direct effect of the lithium but is also due to drinking increased volumes of high-calorie fluids — for example, tea or coffee with sugar, soft drinks, fruit juices and alcoholic beverages. It is best to drink water, mineral water, or tea and coffee without sugar. The small amount of lithium in mineral water will not affect your lithium blood levels.

Less common side-effects are:

- **Nausea:** This can be caused by the tablet partly dissolving in the mouth, or from taking them on an empty stomach. It can often be minimised by swallowing the tablets quickly (whole), one at a time, with a large glass of cold water or milk, and by taking them after meals. If you are still having problems getting the tablets down, and are taking Lithicarb, ask your doctor about changing to the slow-release form, Priadel, as this will often help. Avoid using preparations like Dexsal, Enos, Ural or Citravescent. They do not help relieve the nausea to an appreciable extent, but they do lower the blood lithium level.

- **Lethargy:** This is an unusual complaint for people on lithium. Sometimes it is a true side-effect, but most often it is perceived to occur when lithium stops the rapid minor variations in mood which patients had come to regard as normal before treatment.
- **Skin Changes:** Lithium can occasionally cause or worsen acne, psoriasis and some other skin conditions. Usually your own doctor or a dermatologist can recommend ways of helping this. If you have been taking lithium for some years, you might notice your skin becoming dry and scaly. Frequent application of lanolin-based creams or Calmurid will help prevent this.
- **Thyroid Changes:** Lithium can slow the activity of the thyroid gland, usually after a number of years of lithium therapy. For the majority of people this does not occur; however, most doctors annually check the thyroid function of patients taking lithium. If the thyroid gland has been slowed down, the addition of thyroid supplement tablets to your treatment will correct this problem. The activity of the gland commonly returns to normal if lithium is ceased, and, in any case, treatment of the problem is simple and safe.

Toxic Effects of Lithium

If you take your lithium tablets as prescribed, have regular blood level checks and make sure you quench your thirst in hot weather, then there is little chance of the lithium in your blood reaching a toxic level. However, it is important for you to be aware of the symptoms of toxicity, and to know how to manage them. The most common ways in which people can develop toxicity are by:

- **Becoming dehydrated.** This might occur in very hot weather because of insufficient fluid intake (especially if you are working hard and sweating profusely), or if you lose fluid from your body by other means — for example, vomiting and diarrhoea from gastro-enteritis or food poisoning. If you have gastro-enteritis you should stop your lithium until it has settled, and contact your doctor. (It is most unlikely that you will suffer a relapse of your mood disorder while you are unable to take the lithium medication.)
- **Suddenly reducing your salt intake** — for example, in some diets. Do not radically decrease or increase your salt intake

without contacting your doctor.

- **Taking the wrong dose.** When you are on long-term therapy, it is sometimes easy to forget that you have taken your tablets, and so take a second dose. This should cause toxicity only if you are also dehydrated. It is a good idea to take tablets in association with a routine activity, such as breakfast and going to bed. If you realise you have forgotten a dose after more than four hours, do not take it. No harm will result. When you take your tablets, put a cross on a calendar kept with the bottle, or consider buying a Dosette box from your chemist, so you can keep track. Taking a higher dose than you should is more dangerous for elderly people.
- **Taking other drugs.** Some drugs can cause the blood level of lithium to rise. If another doctor is prescribing any new tablets for you, tell him or her that you are on lithium.

Be particularly aware of diuretics (tablets to get rid of excess fluid — for example, Aprinox (bendrofluazide), Chlotride (chlorothiazide), Dichlotride (hydrochlorothiazide), Enduron (methyclothiazide), Hygroton (chlorthalidone), Moduretic (hydrochlorothiazide with amiloride) and Navidrex (cyclopenthiazide). Not all diuretics affect lithium levels. Also avoid taking tablets for arthritis and pain — for example, Brufen (ibuprofen), Feldene (priroxicam), Indocid (indomethacin), Naprogesic (naproxen sodium), Naprosyn (naproxen), Orudis (ketoprofen), Ponstan (mefenamic acid) and Voltaren (diclofenac).

Symptoms of Toxicity

You might experience any of the following if your blood lithium level becomes toxic:

- Vomiting or severe diarrhoea.
- Severe drowsiness.
- Confusion/severe forgetfulness.
- Severe tremor/shakiness/staggering.
- Because these toxic symptoms include confusion, forgetfulness and drowsiness, it is very important that someone close to you knows the symptoms to watch for (just as it is important that someone monitors mood changes which you might not notice, particularly if you are on a high).

If you develop any of these symptoms you should:

- Stop taking lithium tablets.
- Drink as much fluid as possible — for example, water, fruit juice or mineral water (minimum – 1 litre in 1 hour)
- Contact your doctor immediately, or go to a hospital Emergency Department and tell the staff you might be suffering from lithium toxicity.

Lithium toxicity can be readily treated, but the sooner the better, as it tends to get worse rapidly if untreated.

Remember, most people take lithium for many years with major benefits and very few problems.

Travel

If you are travelling overseas, make sure you have enough lithium tablets to last throughout your trip, with a few extra to allow for travel delays. It is also a good idea to carry a letter from your doctor stating which tablets you are taking and why. This will assist you in obtaining further supplies of tablets should you lose yours, and can save much potential trouble with customs inspectors!

Pregnancy

Although approximately ninety per cent of women taking lithium have normal pregnancies and healthy babies, current medical opinion is that there might be a risk of abnormalities, particularly of the heart, in 5–10 per cent of babies if the mother is taking lithium during the first three months of pregnancy. If you are contemplating becoming pregnant while on lithium, you should discuss this with your doctor.

Major surgery

Lithium does not appear to cause problems with anaesthetics, but lithium toxicity can result from post-operative dehydration. If you have to undergo an operation which requires a general anaesthetic, notify your psychiatrist, who can then speak to the surgeon about adjusting your lithium medication in order to avoid lithium toxicity.

A GUIDE TO MONOAMINE OXIDASE INHIBITORS (MAOIs)

What are monoamine oxidase inhibitors and when are they prescribed?
Monoamine oxidase inhibitors (MAOIs) are a group of drugs which relieve the effects of depressive illness, including agitation and lowered moods. They are also effective in relieving panic attacks and anxiety in some people.

MAOIs available in Australia are: phenelzine (Nardil®), tranylcypromine (Parnate®) and tranylcypromine with trifluoperazine (Parstelin®). They are taken in tablet form. Moclobemide (Aurorix®) is a new MAOI to which some of the advice in this guide does not apply.

How do they work?
MAOIs all act on the brain in a similar manner, partly by altering concentrations of chemicals which transmit signals from one nerve cell to another (neurotransmitters). Although they are mood elevators, they are **not** addictive, as amphetamines ('speed') are.

How soon will I feel better?
The first beneficial effect you can expect is the relief of agitation. The elevating effect on the depressed mood does not usually become apparent for one to three weeks, or more. For this reason it is important not to abandon the treatment through frustration at the presence of side-effects and lack of improvement in the early stages. People in all sorts of jobs tolerate full doses of antidepressants and cope fully with their normal work situations.

If you cease your medication abruptly you might have an unpleasant (though not dangerous) reaction, including dizziness, nausea and diarrhoea, so if you want to give up the treatment, discuss how to do so with your doctor.

How and when do I take the medication?
MAOIs are usually taken early in the day because they tend to cause or increase difficulty in sleeping for most patients. However, some patients experience a sedative effect, and in that case they may be taken at night.

The dose required to relieve symptoms varies greatly depending on each individual's body chemistry. For this reason, and because side-effects are more of a problem when the initial does is high, it is best to commence with a small dose and build up the dose as rapidly as side-effects allow. Your doctor will be seeing you frequently at this stage of your treatment, will discuss the side-effects, and will advise on the rate of increase of the dose. If you are feeling very uncomfortable, contact your doctor.

Interactions with foods, liquor and medications
These drugs might interact with aged protein in food and drink, and with certain drugs, producing a sudden increase in blood pressure and severe headache. Precautions must therefore be taken if you develop a very severe headache seek medical attention immediately. If the headache is due to an increase in blood pressure, an injection of phentolamine (Regitine®) or chlorpromazine (Largactil®), or oral nifedipine (Adalat®), or one of a number of alternative medications, will reduce the blood pressure to normal levels. Take this guide with you in case your doctor is not aware of the name of the antidote.

What side-effects might I experience, and what can I do about them?
Feelings of *dizziness* or *faintness* might occur if you have strenuous exercise, stand for long periods, or change position suddenly. Avoid these actions if possible, and avoid hot baths. If you stand up slowly you will lessen the problem, but if the faintness continues, tell your doctor.

During the first few weeks of taking MAOIS you might experience *dryness of the mouth,* which can be relieved by sips of a low-calorie drink, or by sucking low-calorie jobes or sweets. Other common side-effects are a *fine tremor, constipation, and blurring of vision* when reading small print. Difficulties in reading can be overcome by purchasing over-the-counter glasses. If you are an inpatient, some hospitals provide corrective spectacles to enable you to read or to do fine work.

You might notice a *reduction in sexual response.* Your sex drive might improve with effective treatment of your depression and, in any case will revert to its usual level on ceasing the tablets. You should discuss the problem with your doctor if it is particularly worrying.

If the tablets give you *indigestion,* take them with food or a glass of milk.

If you feel *drowsy* or less alert during the first few weeks, you should be particularly careful about *driving or working with machinery.* If you combine MAOIS with any alcohol, you should not drive a car or operate power tools or machinery. the combination of MAOIS and *alcohol* might have serious effects, and you should be cautious about combining the two drugs.

You might *gain weight.* The amount you gain might be more than any you lost while you were ill (less commonly, some people lose weight). Part of this gain is due to the medication stimulating the appetite for sweet foods, but part might be due to an effect on the body's metabolism. In any case, regular exercise and a sensible diet are the only solutions until you can reduce or cease the medication.

There are other uncommon side-effects. The best advice is to speak to your doctor or pharmacist about any concerns which arise after you begin taking the medication. Side-effects can often be eased by a variety of measures.

All the side-effects mentioned tend to reduce over a period of time, and most people have no problem in resuming their normal occupation once the depression has lifted.

How long do I have to continue taking MAOIs?

Reliable trials assessing the effect of antidepressant treatment have shown that the possiblity of relapse is much less if the medication is continued for at least three months after relief from your depressive illness. As with most medication, the duration of your treatment will vary between individuals, and your doctor will advise you.

It is important to reduce your medication slowly under the guidance of your treating doctor. You might experience vivid dreams during the reduction in dosage, but, as mentioned earlier, MAOIs are not addictive.

If you suffer a relapse, your doctor will discuss with you the pros and cons of longer-term maintenance therapy.

The dangers of overdosing

MAOIs are dangerous if an overdose is taken and particularly dangerous for children. They should be kept in a safe child-proof place. Your doctor might ask you to give them to your partner, if you have one, or to another family member or friend, as a safety precaution.

Medications in this group are sometimes prescribed together with other antidepressants; for example, tricyclic antidepressants. However, precautions should be taken and this is one reason why it is very important to tell a new doctor which medications you are taking.

Travel

Carry two days' supply in your purse or wallet, in case you are unexpectedly away overnight.

If you are travelling overseas, make sure you have enough tablets to last throughout your trip, with a few extra to allow for travel delays. It is also a good idea to carry a letter from your doctor stating which tablets you are taking and why. This will assist you in obtaining further supplies of tablets should you lose yours, and can save much potential trouble with customs inspectors!

Pregnancy

MAOIS have not been shown to be associated with an increased occurrence of birth abnormalities. Ideally, however, pregnancy should be drug free, and your doctor will decide whether there are sound reasons to recommend the use of these medications during a pregnancy.

MAOIs and food

The most important guideline is to avoid any substance which has previously produced unpleasant symptoms, and to discuss any such reaction with your doctor. If in doubt about a food or beverage, consume a teaspoonful on the first occasion. If you have no unpleasant symptoms that day, you can safely try a little more next time. If you consume a small amount of a number of different foods and drinks listed below on the one day, you might exceed the safety limit.

The following foods are likely to produce reactions and should be avoided:

- Cheese: Eighty per cent of adverse reactions involve cheese. Cottage cheese, ricotta cheese, cream cheese, and mild processed cheese are safe. However, the rule about a trial sample mentioned above should be followed, and you are advised not to eat aged or ripened cheese.

- Salami (especially uncooked, smoked salami), air-dried sausage, prosciutto.
- Meat and yeast extract, such as Marmite®, Vegemite®, Promite® and Bonox®.
- Packaged soups or stock cubes.
- Any of the following products if stale: meat, fish, poultry, game, offal, pate, yoghurt, cream. (Stale meat does not mean cooked meats, such as ham, corned beef, and so on, but meats that have been aged or stored for a long time or smell 'off'.)
- Chiko Rolls and Dim Sims, which sometimes contain quite aged meat products.
- Smoked or pickled fish; caviar; tarama and taramasalata.
- Sauerkraut, broad bean pods, banana skins, and any processed banana-flavoured foods; for example, yoghurt and chips (whole bananas are often emulsified to provide flavouring in these products).
- Over-ripe avocado.
- Coffee substitutes; for example, Ecco coffee.
- Fermented soy bean products; for example, tofu.

Note: Condiments and herbs are not dangerous.

Eating out

Check with the provider that there is no cheese in the dish, and avoid heavy sauces.

MAOIs and migraine

Chocolate and strong percolated coffee might trigger a migraine-like headache in people taking MAOIs, but they do not cause high blood pressure.

MAOIs and alcohol

Don't drink home-brewed beer or liqueurs.

Spirits do not cause the high-blood-pressure reaction. Do not consume more than three standard drinks of any other alcoholic beverage in one day.

In addition to the high-blood-pressure reaction already mentioned, any alcoholic drink might interact with prescribed and over-the-counter medicines and produce unpleasant side-effects.

MAOIS and drugs

Patients taking MAOIS should consult their doctor or pharmacist before taking any other medications, including over-the-counter products. This includes cough and cold remedies and pain killers. Aspirin and Paracetamol are safe in the recommended doses. Inform your dentist that you are taking an MAOI.

Tryptophan is an aminoacid which is an ingredient of a normal diet. However, when taken as a medication in combination with MAOIs, it has been reported to cause adverse reactions, including manic excitement. It is advisable to speak to your psychiatrist before taking it.

MAOIs and diabetes

If you are diabetic and on anti-diabetic agents you might need to reduce your dose of diabetic medication. Discuss this with your doctor.

Precautions after ceasing MAOIs

MAOIs remain in the body for a considerable time after the medication is ceased. In order to avoid the risk of a reaction when the drug is no longer being taken, it is wise to continue the diet for two weeks.

Important DOs and DON'Ts

DO follow the advice about interactions with food, alcohol, and medication.

DO tell any doctor you consult what medications you are taking.

DO persist with the medication for at least a month if possible.

DO report any worrying symptoms that develop after starting the medication — not just the side-effects mentioned in this guide.

DO tell your doctor if you intend to become pregnant.

DON'T combine the medication with alcohol, then drive or use machinery.

DON'T stop your medication suddenly.

DON'T take a double dose if you have forgotten the last one and the next dose is due within four hours.

Which advice should you follow?

You might read other advice sheets containing different dietary and medication instructions for people taking MAOIS. Some include warnings about substances which we consider safe and have not included. We believe our advice is based on the most up-to-date and reliable information but, if you are in doubt, discuss the matter with your doctor.

All of the information in this appendix is available in brochure form from The Melbourne Clinic, 130 Church Street, Richmond, Victoria 3121.

Appendix IV

A GUIDE TO TRICYCLIC ANTIDEPRESSANTS

What are tricyclic antidepressants and when are they prescribed?

Tricyclic antidepressants are a group of medications used to treat the effects of depressive illness, which include agitation, insomnia, lowered mood, loss of energy and interest, and feelings of guilt.

Included in this family of medications are amitriptyline (Tryptanol®, Laroxyl®, Endep®, Amitrip®, Saroten®), clomipramine (Anafranil®) desipramine (Pertofran®), dothiepin (Prothiaden®), doxepin (Sinequan®, Deptran®), imipramine (Tofranil®), nortriptyline (Allegron®, Nortab®) and trimipramine (Surmontil®). (Some of these are also used for the treatment of obsessive-compulsive disorder, phobic anxiety and other anxiety disorders.) They are usually in tablet or capsule form, but some are available as a syrup.

How do they work?

Tricyclic antidepressants all act on the brain in a similar manner, partly by altering concentrations of chemicals which transmit signals from one nerve cell to the next (neurotransmitters). Tricyclic antidepressants are not stimulants like amphetamine ('speed') or caffeine, and are **not** addictive.

How soon will I feel better?

The first beneficial effect you can expect is the relief of agitation and insomnia. The elevating effect on the depressed mood does not usually become apparent for one to three weeks, or more. For this eason it is important not to abandon the treatment through frustration at the lack of improvement in the early stages. People in all sorts of jobs tolerate full doses of antidepressants and cope fully with their normal work situations.

If you cease your medication abruptly you might have an unpleasant (though not dangerous) reaction, including dizziness, nausea and diarrhoea, so if you want to give up the treatment discuss how to do so with your doctor.

How and when do I take the medication?
Tricyclic antidepressants are usually taken at night, because they have a sedative effect which helps relieve the insomnia that is common in major depression. They stay in the body for a longer time than some other medications and so they do not need to be taken at regular intervals during the day; once a day is sufficient. They are best taken an hour or so before you go to bed, the exact time depending on how long they take to make you sleepy. If they should happen to aggravate sleeplessness, then take them in the morning.

The dose required to relieve symptoms varies greatly, depending on each individual's body chemistry, from (rarely) one 25-mg tablet or capsule to twelve or more. For this reason, and because side-effects are more of a problem when the initial dose is high, it is best to commence with a small dose at night and build up the dose as rapidly as side-effects allow. Your doctor will be seeing you frequently at this stage of your treatment and will discuss the side-effects and advise on the rate of increase of the dose. If you are very uncomfortable, contact your doctor.

If you forget a night does, you might be reminded of it by restlessness. If this happens less than eight hours after it was due, take it but remember that you will probably be sleepy during the following day. Similarly, a dose of a drug which alerts you might cause insomnia that night if taken in the afternoon.

What side-effects might I experience, and what can I do about them?
Dryness of the mouth nearly always occurs and some people notice a peculiar tast. The dryness can be relieved by sips of a low calorie drink, or by sucking low-calorie sweets. Low-calorie products help in weight management (see page 67).

Many people experience undue sleepiness or a 'drugged' feeling in the first few days. This usually wears off; if it doesn't, speak to your doctor, who will either adjust the dosage or change you to another less sedating tricyclic medication.

Other common side-effects are a *slight tremor, palpitation, constipation,* and *dizziness* on standing up. The dizziness can be minimised by avoiding very hot baths and by standing up slowly. If it persists, speak to your doctor, who might suggest other measures to reduce the problems. Another side-effect is *blurring of vision* when reading small print, and you might find it worthwhile to purchase corrective over-the-counter glasses. If you are an inpatient, some hospitals provide corrective spectacles to enable you to read or to do fine work.

You might notice a *reduction in sexual response.* Your sex drive might improve with effective treatment of your depression and, in any case, will revert to its usual level on ceasing the medication. You should discuss the problem with your doctor if it is particularly worrying.

If the tablets give you *indigestion,* take them with food or a glass of milk.

For people who suffer from *epilepsy, glaucoma* or *heart* disease or who are receiving certain medications for *high* blood pressure, treatment with tricyclic antidepressants might mean that these medications need to be adjusted. If you suffer any of these conditions you should ensure that the doctor prescribing the antidepressant medication is aware of the fact, as he or she might wish to consult with the other doctors treating you.

You might *gain weight.* The amount you gain might be more than any you lost while you were ill. Part of this gain is due to the medication stimulating the appetite for sweet foods, but part might be due to an effect on the body's metabolism. In any case, regular exercise and a sensible diet are the only solutions until you can reduce or cease the medication.

There are other uncommon side-effects. The best advice is to speak to your doctor or pharmacist about any concerns which arise after you begin taking the medication. Side-effects can often be eased by a variety of measures.

As with almost all medications used for emotional and mental disorders, if you *combine antidepressants and any alcohol* you should not drive a car or operate power tools or machinery. Some people become very ill combining antidepressants and alcohol, and if you combine the two you should do so cautiously. Taking entidepressants will not usually interfere with your ability to drive a vehicle or operate machinery once you have adjusted to the side-effects.

All the side-effects mentioned tend to reduce over a period

of time, and most people have no problem in resuming their normal occupation once the depression has lifted.

How long do I have to continue taking tricyclic antidepressants?

Reliable trials assessing the effect of tricyclic antidepressant treatment have shown that the possibility of relapse is much less if the medication is continued for at least three months after relief from your depressive illness. As with most medication, the duration of your treatment will vary between individuals and your doctor will advise you.

It is important to reduce your medication slowly under the guidance of your treating doctor. You might experience vivid dreams during the reduction in dosage but, as mentioned earlier, tricyclic antidepressants are not addictive.

If you suffer a relapse your doctor will discuss with you the pros and cons of longer term maintenance therapy.

Special Precautions

Tricyclic antidepressants are dangerous if an overdose is taken, and particularly dangerous for children. They should be kept in a safe child-proof place. Your doctor might ask you to give them to your partner, if you have one, or other family member or friend as a safety precaution.

Medications in this group are sometimes prescribed together with other antidepressants; for example, monoamine oxidase inhibitors. However, precautions are usually required and this is one reason why it is very important to tell a new doctor which medications you are taking.

Travel

Carry two days' supply in your purse or wallet, in case you are unexpectedly away overnight.

If you are travelling overseas, make sure you have enough tablets to last throughout your trip, with a few extra to allow for travel delays. It is also a good idea to carry a letter from your doctor stating which tablets you are taking and why. This will assist you in obtaining further supplies of tablets should you lose yours, and can save much potential trouble with customs inspectors!

Pregnancy

Tricyclic antidepressants have not been shown to be associated with an increased occurrence of birth abnormalities. Ideally, however, pregnancy should be drug free, and your doctors will decide whether there are sound reasons to recommend the use of these medications during a pregnancy.

Important DOs and DON'Ts

DO tell any doctor you consult what medications you are taking.
DO persist with the medication for at least a month if possible.
DO report any worrying symptoms that develop after starting the medication – not just the side-effects mentioned in this guide.
DO tell your doctor if you intend to become pregnant.
DON'T combine the medication with alcohol, then drive or use machinery.
DON'T stop your medication suddenly.
DON'T take a double dose if you have forgotten the last one and the next dose is due.

All of the information in this appendix is available in brochure form from The Melbourne Clinic, 130 Church Street, Richmond, Victoria 3121.

Appendix V

GROUPS AND ASSOCIATIONS

Self-help Groups

A.C.T.

Canberra Manic-depressive Support Group
Pat Daniels
28 Paloona Place
DUFFY ACT 2611
(062) 88 2747

New South Wales

Manda Newcastle Organisation
15 Hudson Street
HAMILTON NSW 2303
John Nesbitt
(049) 61 4984

Northern Beaches Manic-depressive Self-help Group
Tony Francis Kalayzich
17 Pacific Parade
DEE WHY NSW 2099
Iris Hardcastle
(02) 982 9155

Phil
26 Llandaff Street
BONDI JUNCTION NSW
(02) 519 5286

Sydney Manic-depressive Self-help Group
Meg Smith
41 Ilka Street
LILYFIELD NSW 2040
H (02) 660 7413
W (02) 772 9200
–299

New Zealand

Manic Depressive Society
Mr Chris Howison
PO Box 25.068
CHRISTCHURCH NZ

Kerry Hand
Director
Social and Rehabilitation Centre
9 Union Street
DUNEDIN NZ

Queensland

Ipswich MD Group
John Hildebrand
17 Hayden Street
RIVERVIEW QLD 4304
(07) 282 3781

Manic-Depressive Support Group (Brisbane)
'Friendship House'
20 Balfour Street
NEW FARM QLD 4005
W (07) 358 4988

Moodswing Illness Prevention
Suzanne Wootton
C/- Townsville Women's Centre
50 Patrick Street
AITKENVALE QLD 4814
(077) 75 7555

South Australia

Angela Mandary
Murray Mallee Community Health Service
Edmond Crossing House
18 Beatie Terrace
MURRAY BRIDGE SA 5253
(085) 32 6088

Judy Schroeder
Co-ordinator
Pinnaroo 'Hub Neighbourhood House'
Bundy Terrace
PINNAROO SA 3304
(085) 77 8485

Victoria

Cheltenham Group
Pam Houston
Cheltenham Neighbourhood House
8 Chesterville Road
CHELTENHAM VIC 3192
H (03) 553 4163
W (03) 583 0095

Geelong Bi-polar Support Group
C/- Wayne Casey
218 Ryrie Street
GEELONG VIC 3220
(052) 26 7490

MDP Support Group
Ian Eames
9 Nilmar Avenue
WODONGA VIC 3690
(060) 56 1700

Moodswing Group
Judith Player
615 Camberwell Road
CAMBERWELL VIC 3124
(03) 889 3733

Warrnambool Moodswing Support Group
Ken Burnett 'Alveston'
76 Banyan Street
WARRNAMBOOL VIC 3280
(055) 62 4188

Mental Health Associations

A.C.T.
Mental Health Foundation (ACT)
Level 5 Tower Building
ACTON ACT 2601
(06) 247 5861

New South Wales
NSW Association for Mental Health
63 Victoria Road
GLADESVILLE NSW 2111
(02) 816 1611

New Zealand
Mental Health Foundation of New Zealand
PO Box 37– 438 Parnell
272 Parnell Road
AUCKLAND 1
303 1517

Northern Territory
NT Association for Mental Health
PO Box 1370
DARWIN NT 0801

Queensland
Qld Association for Mental Health
Friendship House
20 Balfour Street
NEWFARM QLD 4005
(07) 358 4988

South Australia

Mental Health Association & Resource Centre (SA) Inc
35 Fullarton Road
KENT TOWN SA 5067
(08) 362 6772

Tasmania

Tas Association for Mental Health
PO Box 235
NORTH HOBART TAS 7100
(002) 78 1557

Victoria

Mental Health Foundation of Australia
1 Cookson Street
CAMBERWELL VIC 3124
(03) 813 2848

Mental Health Foundation (Victoria)
1 Cookson Street
CAMBERWELL VIC 3124
(03) 813 3736

Western Australia

WA Association for Mental Health
2 Nicholson Street
SUBIACO WA 6008
(09) 381 1986

Appendix VI

BOOKS FOR THE JOURNEY

Branden, N, *How to Raise Your Self-esteem,* Bantam, USA, 1988
A pocket book with a fund of commonsense items and exercises to build self-esteem, which is deficient in most of us. Even if a person's self-esteem has been reasonably adequate before bouts of mania and depression, it is one of the areas of personality which takes a beating afterwards.

Bruckne-Gordon, F, *Making Therapy Work,* Harper & Row, USA, 1988
A much-needed lay-level book helping people to choose doctors and therapists, and decide what they hope to gain, how to work through difficulties with a therapist, and when to terminate treatment. Ideal for anyone working with psychiatrists or other therapists.

Clairborne-Park, C, *You Are Not Alone,* Atlantic Little Brown, USA, 1976
A book which describes the effect of living with mental illness and its impact on spouses, relatives, and friends. Describes common experiences and how to deal with them.

Fieve, R, *Moodswings,* Bantam, USA, 1976
A colourful presentation of mood swings, famous sufferers and lithium as a revolutionary treatment. Illuminating chapters on creativity and psychotherapy. Written by a psychiatrist who specialises in treating mood swings.

Herman, N, *Why Psychotherapy?* Free Association Books, 1987
An accessible description of the process of dynamic psychotherapy. Also highly critical of a purely medical approach to human suffering.

Kuipers, L, *Living with Mental Illness,* Condor, UK, 1987
An excellent work assisting families to come to terms with psychiatric problems. It suggests ways of handling all people — those who are hyperactive, paranoid, depressed, or delusional. A book many families will identify with.

McCallum, P, *A Family in Therapy,* McPhee Gribble, Melbourne, 1980
A sensitive account of a family in therapy.

McKeon, P, *Coping with Depression and Elation,* Sheridan Press London 1986
A comprehensive and practical guide to causes, treatment, alternative strategies, and genetics. Questions chapter very useful.

MacNab, F, *Change,* Hill of Content, Melbourne, 1984
Typical of Dr MacNab's works, this is realistic, practical and sensitive. People with bipolar disorder go through enormous change, and reading this book can be a comfort and a guide.

MacNab, F, *Coping,* Hill of Content, Melbourne, 1985
Covers skills, strategies and resources required to cope with stress situations. Includes ways of dealing with stress.

Scott Peck, M, *The Road Less Travelled,* Rider, London, 1988
Written by a spiritual psychiatrist, this work focusses attention on taking responsibility for ourselves, and change and how this affects our relationships. Good for people who have separation, divorce or finding another mate on their minds.

Russianoff, P, *When Am I Going to Be Happy?* Bantam, USA, 1988
All mood swing sufferers at some stage have to learn to surmount self-pity and strive for an attitude or philosophy regarding happiness. This book could serve as an aid.

Ryan, R S & Travis, J W, *Wellness Workbook,* Ten Speed Press, USA, 1981
A wholistic approach to health and personal growth which can help you deal with grief, anger, and assertion. Again, its aim is to motivate the reader to accept responsibility and the choices available for optimum health.

Williams, N, *Rekindling Desire,* New Harbinger Publishers, California, 1988
A gentle book, helping people to restore or enrich their sexual lives. It may be useful for partners with sexual half- heartedness following bouts of depression or manic promiscuity and excessive demands.

Schou, M, *Lithium Treatment of Manic-depressive Illness,* Karger, Switzerland, 1978
Extremely useful information and advice. A practical guide providing answers to the many questions manic depression sufferers will have.

Yalon, I D, *Love's Executioner,* Basic Books, New York, 1989
Beautifully written tales of psychotherapeutic encounters by a gifted therapist.

INDEX